It’s Not OK To Be Not OK

It's Not OK To Be Not

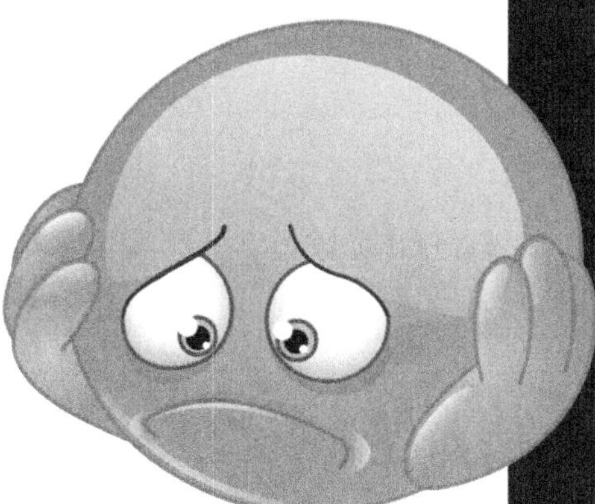

K

HOW TO STOP THE WORLD SCREWING WITH YOUR HEAD

STUART WELBOURN

Reality Responsibility Publishing

ISBN: 978-1-0684175-0-4 (Paperback)

ISBN: 978-1-0684175-1-1 (eBook)

Disclaimer

The author of this book does not dispense medical advice or prescribe the use of any technique as treatment for physical or mental health conditions without the advice of a qualified physician, either directly or indirectly. The intent of the author is to offer information to help you with your search for better well-being only. In the event you use any of the information in this book for yourself, the author and the publisher assume no responsibility for your actions.

For Chris and Stuart,

They departed too soon but will always be remembered.

Contents

Preface

Yes, you read the book title correctly—it's not a typo. I mean it when I say, "It's Not OK to be Not OK." While well-meaning, the phrase "It's OK to be Not OK" or similar variations no longer serve the same beneficial purpose as when they were first shared publicly. The earliest example I could find online dates back to a blog post from 2013. It may have been used before then. However, the widespread use of the term online did not occur until a few years later. It has become one of those clichéd buzz phrases now uttered with normality rather than genuine emotion. A little bit like when someone says "there, there" as a form of comfort. But like many of these modern never thought through fully ideas and tropes, it has begun to grit my shit when I see or hear it.

When I searched on Amazon, I found 536 T-shirts with various designs, including variants such as "It's OK Not to Be OK" printed on the front, and thousands of posters and badges. There were also forty-five books published since 2018 that contain the phrase in their title, most of which seem to offer mental health support, although I have not read any of them. Whether these books are any good, I cannot say, but my attack is on the phrase and not against these authors.

Just like with advertising, when we hear a message often enough, it becomes embedded in our subconscious. For example, if I were to say, "Because you're worth it," you would probably know what product uses this in its advertising. I know it, and I rarely watch adverts. Plus, I haven't needed to use hair products for over two decades. The world is constantly bombarding us with messages, and most of them are screwing with our heads in some way or another. They are all designed to manipulate us to think or feel a certain way. Some are designed to benefit us, but most don't fall into that category, but this isn't always by design. This is why we must be careful with what phrases we associate with our health.

Let me explain: words hold specific meanings in our subconscious, and we often interpret them literally. If the phrase were "It's OK to 'FEEL' not OK", I may not have found the need to write this book, although I would still like to add the word "sometimes" before "feel". But no, it's to "BE" not OK, which concerns me with regard to improving mental health. What does it mean to be something? In its most accurate sense, it is about whom or what something is at all times. To be a dog, one has to be a dog, and it will always be so for the dog; a dog can never "BE" a cat. If you are not a dog, you can only guess what it is like to be one.

It's important to understand that "being" not OK can be seen by some as a permanent condition, and it appears that an increasing number of people are accepting this as the norm. There will be those who may argue I am splitting hairs over semantics, but based on what I see, if I'm wrong, no harm will come to those who choose to ditch this phrase. However, if I'm right, this saying now does more harm than good, but I'll let you decide by reading this book to the end. If you currently find the phrase comforting in any way, remember that this is nowhere near as comforting as getting an issue fully resolved. At the same time, how insulting is it to say to someone born with a permanent condition that they are not OK?

In my opinion, there is a lot of stuff posted online to do with mental health, which is, quite frankly, a load of bollocks. I won't be specific, as that would probably land me in the shit. What I have to say may well be bollocks too, but I do not feel so. I certainly do not expect you to believe anything I share in this book. By the time it's published and the first copies are sold, there will probably be bits I disagree with or could improve upon. Typically, I listen to one new audiobook each week focused on psychology, philosophy, and related topics. As a result, I frequently gain new insights from this study. Being rigid in your beliefs does no good, especially when presented with reliable and contradictory new data. The information presented here draws from statistical and academic research, personal training, observation, experience, and some current subjective conclusions derived from this data.

As with everything in life, I advise people to conduct research and not believe anything unquestioningly. We now live in a time where pretty much anything can be made to appear genuine, and discerning what is true from what is false is beyond the abilities of most of us. Many individuals often think that only the ideas they oppose are false, while viewing anything that aligns with their beliefs as true. There are also far too many people who believe and share any old shit that's posted online or printed in a tabloid. This is why I also encourage people to maintain an open mind and incorporate as much humour into their lives as possible; more on that later.

Let me clarify one thing before we go any further: if you are not feeling OK for whatever reason, there is nothing wrong with you. You are not broken, and there are ways for you to feel OK again, which I will also discuss. I sincerely want you to finish reading this book with the hope that there is a way to improve things, no matter how bad you or someone you care about currently feels.

I may be blunt at times, but not all therapy involves being "nice"; sometimes, a client needs to be pushed through something painful to come out the other side far stronger, essentially going from "victim" to "victor". Knowing when to use this approach and when not to takes training, experience, and maybe a little bit of intuition. However, my ability to assist through a book is limited compared to personalised, one-on-one interactions. I wish to avoid causing anyone additional distress, so I won't be too rough.

Obtaining the specific support you may need is beyond any book's scope, but I will provide some pointers on what to look for and avoid. My first tip would be to avoid seeking advice from what I call "narci-chologists" who promote a single idea as "the only solution", with the additional view that all other approaches have got it wrong. There's another term for those who are so convinced that everyone else is mistaken; it's arrogant. This is not to say their technique doesn't work, but what works for one person may not work for another. A phrase which has always stuck with me since I first started training as a therapist is “horses for courses”. It was pointed out early on that Hypnoanalysis can help with many conditions, but it isn’t a panacea. Nothing I am aware of is a cure-all; there will always be someone for whom a technique does not work.

I find it an interesting coincidence that a word I created by blending "narcissist" and "psychologist," when spoken aloud, sounds almost like "Nazi-chologist." The Nazis were singularly minded, and you wouldn’t want to take advice from one, would you? So, this might be a way to remember this in the future when seeking help. I should point out that I do not work as a therapist at the moment, so I am not trying to sell you any of my services. In my opinion, a good therapist prioritises the client and should suggest alternative techniques if their methods are not achieving the desired result. They should also recommend a competent professional if they know one, but hey, that’s just me.

I will not be using lots of psychology jargon or going too deep into the points I shall be making, but instead, I will try to keep explanations short and straightforward to avoid confusion or overwhelm. Plenty of books and articles are already available if you want to go deep into the topic of mental health. But fair warning, if you choose to go down that rabbit hole, you’ll eventually realise it has no exit. I’ve been tunnelling away for three decades and barely got beneath this fascinating subject's surface.

Additional warning; if you do not like strong language, put the book down now and either give it to charity or someone who might benefit from it who swears like a fucking sailor. If you don’t mind most swear words except one in particular, let me assure you, I will not be using the “C” word at any point. I’m not using profanity to come across as cool or edgy like some do, and I won't be overusing it. But, sometimes, a swear word conveys a point far better than an articulate alternative. Mostly, I'll use it to amuse myself, and hopefully, you too, because if you're going to spend hours a day for weeks typing about mental health, you need a bit of light relief. Also, I am an ex-fucking sailor, so what do you fucking expect!

During my research, it was suggested that instead of using the word "suffering," which might be considered insensitive regarding poor mental health, the term "diagnosed" should be used. Since the vast majority of people do not get a formal diagnosis, I will disregard this suggestion in this book. I have suffered from poor mental health and was also diagnosed; neither word had any bearing on how I felt.

If you find anything offensive in this book, that feeling is all yours and has nothing to do with the words themselves. Anything of significance, written or spoken, will offend somebody somewhere. If it doesn't upset anyone, then it's just bland, forgettable nonsense. If I don't say at least one thing which annoys every single reader of this book, then I have failed, even though that is not my real intention. But if you do feel like this at any point, here's a gentle reminder: this self-help book was created to encourage you to reflect on ways to enhance your mental health. That was my heartfelt intention right from the moment I began writing it. How you respond to it is beyond my control, but every single sentence has been given serious contemplation to be included, even the ones which could unintentionally hurt somebody's feelings or seem irrelevant.

As I discuss many common behaviours that I believe indicate some level of poor mental health, you may find that you identify with one or more of these traits. So, by the time you get to the end of the book, you may be inclined to think of me as a bit of a judgmental prick. While that's perfectly fine if you do, you're free to think of me in any way you wish; it's none of my business, but I would like to clarify that I am simply commenting on a particular type of behaviour. When a negative characteristic is pointed out to us, we may be more motivated to change it. If no one ever points it out, we remain oblivious and carry on as usual. Of course, some will still carry on regardless. Let me make it clear, though, that if there is any judgment from me, it is purely on the deed and not on the person. We all have shit going on, and sometimes we can be a bit of a twat, but there are other times when we can be truly astounding. We all make mistakes, which we hopefully learn from, so defining a person by a single action seems like an overreaction to me, generally speaking, of course.

From my perspective as the writer, the best way to read this book is to imagine you're chatting with someone you know while having a brew or possibly a few pints. Perhaps not a close friend, but rather a good acquaintance. Most people know a harmless weirdo who may be a little eccentric yet seems to know a fair bit about many strange topics. You know them well enough to relax in their presence, forgive an occasional faux pas, and recognise they only have your best interests at heart. I am one of those weirdos, so if you didn't know one already, you do now.

I wrote this book with the goal of supporting you on your journey to well-being. I want it to help lessen the extent to which the world screws with your head!

1

Good Intentions Are Not Enough

The internet offers many great benefits, but one downside is that anyone can post anything they want without fully considering the consequences, even though their intentions may be benign.

These days, much of what I see shared is excessively critical and damaging, often neglecting to consider the consequences. We see this all the time with public figures whose posts from years ago resurface to bite them on the ass. While it may have been said innocently and without malice, it can often destroy a person's credibility and even end their career. I find it a strange quirk of human behaviour that, for a social species like ours, we delight in seeing someone fail, especially if we perceive that person to be doing better than us. Everybody gossips and criticises things occasionally, but others make it a full-time career.

Generally speaking, I agree with what Voltaire had to say in *Candide* about the professional critic:

> "A good-for-nothing sort of a man," answered the Abbé, "one who gets his livelihood by abusing every new book and play; he abominates to see anyone meet with success, like eunuchs, who detest everyone that possesses those powers they are deprived of; he is one of those vipers in literature who nourish themselves with their own venom; a pamphlet-monger."[1]

Do you think I intended to come across as sounding cultured and sophisticated by quoting Voltaire? Did I fail miserably and merely sound annoyingly pretentious? A few readers may think the former, probably more the latter, because we are all uniquely different in our tastes. But here's the truth: I used a quote related to my current point to lead into my next one. For the record, I only read a collection of Voltaire's works because he was mentioned several times in the TV series *Sharpe*, starring Sean Bean, and I wanted to know what all the fuss was about.[2] To be fair, I was pleased that I chose to satisfy my curiosity, and I may read some more of his work in the future.

Anyway, I digress; we often face the false dichotomy of selecting between only two perspectives. But, as this simple anecdote illustrates, the absolute truth may lie beyond these options, possibly outside anything which might have crossed your mind. Just a little something to consider when the choices being presented to you make you feel a strong negative emotion. Buying into the "for or against" mentality is too easy to succumb to, so please be mindful of that variety of messaging.

But back to critics, not all do it for money. It is far easier to destroy than to create; however, there is a distinction between pointing out things which can potentially cause harm and being in a constant state of loathing. The first principle in Dale Carnegie's *How to Win Friends and Influence People* is "Do not criticise, condemn, or complain", and those who master this idea tend to have better mental health.[3] So, at this early stage of our journey together, I'd like you to spare a moment to consider how much time you spend on these damaging activities. I haven't completely mastered this idea, but most of my thoughts along these lines do not make it to any kind of public announcement, which is progress. As an exercise, imagine you are incapable of criticising, condemning, or complaining for just one day and see what that turns out like.

Even those with good intentions can inadvertently cause harm with what they share online because they did not think it through thoroughly. I recently shared a brief video on my personal Facebook page, which provided detailed instructions on how to respond to the question posed to test this notion. The instructions were simple; any answer to the question other than "yes" was a "no". This was the question: "Is the phrase 'sharing is caring' positive?" About 80% of respondents said yes, 15% said no, and the remainder didn't follow the instructions.

I think it's great that so many people's first thought came from a heart-centred place. Still, as I hadn't provided any context to the question, it illustrates how many people do not pass their opinions through a reflective brain-centred filter. I must admit that I tried to influence people's answers by mentioning that it was for research for this book on mental health. So, although I hadn't directly given context to the question, some would have assumed the question was related to mental health, sharing problems, etc. Obviously, the saying is neutral until context and positionality are applied. For example, if you had just had sex for the first time with a new partner and they subsequently informed you that they have herpes, you wouldn't consider sharing to be caring, would you?

My little experiment wasn't conducted under scientific conditions with a control group or anything else required for a professional study, so don't take my conclusions as gospel. It would seem that when people think they are being helpful, few give it any more thought or weigh up possible consequences. This is where online advice can become potentially dangerous.

An example of this comes from 2015, called "the black spot campaign". The idea shared by the creators was that if someone was suffering domestic abuse, they could draw a black dot on their palm and secretly use this as a signal to authorities. This sounds like a great idea, in principle, until you give it a little deeper thought. One problem was that the authorities were unaware of the campaign. However, the more concerning aspect that had not been considered was that if it went viral, the perpetrators of such acts would also become aware of the code. There were no reported incidents of harm caused by following this idea, but this doesn't mean they didn't occur; let's hope not. Nevertheless, there were people still sharing the idea on personal websites as recently as 2023.

A similar idea was shared during the COVID-19 lockdowns. In this instance, the idea was to make a phone call pretending to order makeup. Once again, victimisers could become aware of the idea once it had been shared sufficiently. I would also assume that it would have seemed out of place to order makeup at a time when you were only allowed to leave the house for essential purposes and had to wear a mask when you did so. I shared another short video to ask whether women still bothered to wear makeup during this time. I didn't get a large enough response to provide any statistics; some said they did, but more respondents said they didn't. It is still enough to show that this was another idea which sounds great at first until you think about it a little deeper.

This non-thinking attitude to what is shared online is widespread on many topics, but when it is connected with regard to mental health, it can clearly cause harm to some. This is one of the many reasons I say, "It's Not Ok to be Not OK".

2

The Fucking Big Elephant

Normalising poor mental health is fraught with so many potential dangers that I find it unbelievable that I need to point out what is blatantly obvious, the proverbial elephant in the room, or more accurately, the fucking big elephant on the planet. Tune into the news at any time of day or night to be instantly reminded of the dangers associated with poor mental health. This can take many forms, from major incidents to celebrity suicides.

On this last point, it's staggering to think of the number of people each year, famous or not, who get to such a low point that the only option that makes any sense to them is to end their lives. Having that much inner turmoil and believing you have exhausted all your options is one of the lowest points a human can reach. Although I once reached a point where I seriously considered it, I would not even contemplate it now. When you're that depressed, finding a reason to live can be virtually impossible, but finding some reasons not to die may be easier. In my situation, I thought about the fact that I was medically discharged from the Royal Navy and, therefore, will receive a small pension for life. I'll be damned if I'm going to save the Government from paying this out for as long as possible. This is probably not your situation, so you can't really copy this idea exactly, should you ever reach that low point in life. However, the underlying structure of this idea is that you wouldn't want someone or something to benefit from your early demise.

Considering the emotional impact on the person who finds you or the people closest to you may motivate you to keep going. However, the best thing you can do is talk to someone about how you are feeling, which is usually easier if it's a stranger. There are charities with people ready to take your call in this situation, so it's worth giving it a go. It can't hurt to try one last thing, can it?

Most people I have ever spoken to on this subject know someone who took their own life or, at the very least, tried to. In nearly every case, it was unexpected and surprised everyone. I have had two friends end their lives prematurely. One took his life at the height of summer using nitrous oxide and was not found until the smell from his rotting corpse affected his neighbours. His remains were in such a bad state that his mother was not allowed to identify him, and she was a paramedic. What was the reason for this tragic ending, you may be wondering? Well, the straw that broke the proverbial camel's back was over a long-running dispute with the council about his accommodation not being suitable for his extremely rare medical condition. They basically threatened him with some sanctions for saying to them, when totally exasperated, that he may as well save them all the hassle and kill himself! He called their bluff, I guess, and his family have been pursuing this failure in duty of care.

When I was twenty-five, my other friend came out for a few drinks on my stag night. We had no idea he had come for one last drink with his friends before going to a country lane and connecting a hose to his exhaust pipe. To this day, I do not know why he did it. Two young lives were snuffed out before they could reach their potential simply because they did not know where to turn. So, no, it's not OK to BE Not OK. The following three charts will illustrate the severity of this more than any words I can write.

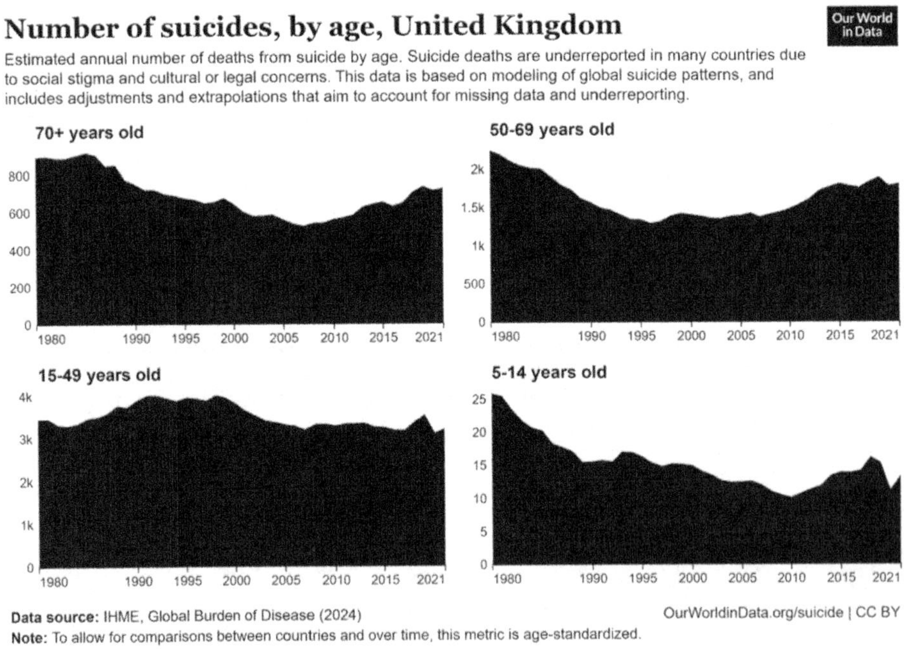

Chart 1 – UK

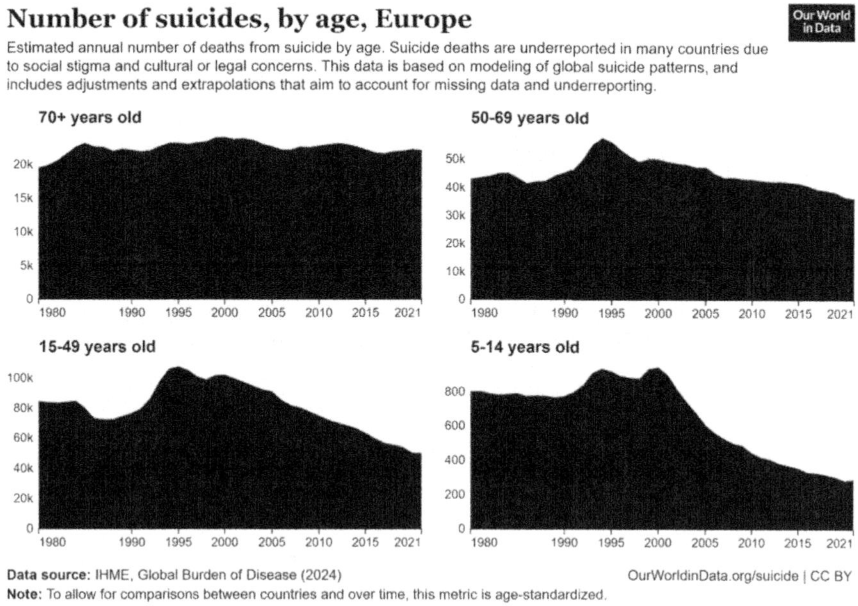

Chart 2

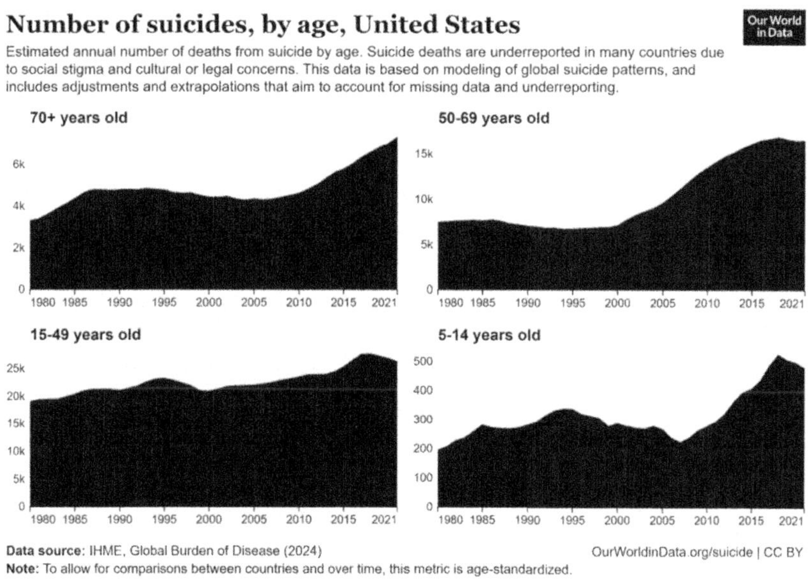

Chart 3 – USA

Charts 1 to 3: IHME, Global Burden of Disease (2024) – with minor processing by Our World in Data.[4]

As tragic as suicide is, generally speaking, the only person who suffers actual physical harm is the person who takes their life. Unfortunately, as we all know too well, people with poor mental health take it out on others.

Mentally healthy people do not pick up assault rifles and kill loved ones or total strangers in a civilian setting. According to the Gun Violence Archive, in 2021, there were 689 mass shootings in the United States; that's almost two a day.[5] What is more distressing is that 327 of these happened at a school, resulting in 81 deaths and 269 injuries, according to USAFacts.org.[6] Here in the U.K., in a similar period, there were 69 homicide victims aged 13 to 19 years; of these, 51 were killed by a knife or sharp instrument, according to the Office for National Statistics.[7]

Some will argue that banning guns and knives will solve the problem, but a mentally unhealthy person determined to carry out homicide will easily find an alternative weapon. It would be impossible to ban everything which can be used to kill another person. This said, a bit of control won't hurt either. You don't need a *Rambo* survival knife or mini-gun to get through the average day.[8]

What constitutes poor mental health ranges from the attention-seeker on social media who believes the world owes them something and should make allowances solely for them to the perpetrators of the most heinous crimes imaginable and everything in between. As a therapist, I have listened as victims of traumatic events have relived these experiences, and I've had to switch off my own emotions to enable me to remain composed and professional to provide the help they needed. It certainly wasn't easy at the beginning of my therapeutic career, and some of the client stories still disturb my thoughts occasionally. It's a burden you must bear, but knowing that clients have found a resolution and can move on with their lives free from the stresses that once troubled them makes it all worthwhile. Yeah, before you say it, being paid is nice, too, but I've probably given just as much of my time helping others for free.

At the other end of the spectrum, after the release of my last book, I spoke to incarcerated Military Veterans who had committed the most despicable of these acts, some against children. It is no easy thing to give up your first inclination to judge a sexual offender as a monster, I can assure you. They know how they are perceived by society and what other prisoners would do if ever able to get their hands on them. Two things still enable me to treat them as human beings. Firstly, in most cases, there is the knowledge that something went wrong for this person in the past, which affected their viewpoint to the extent that they genuinely believed their behaviour was justified. This does not excuse their actions; it just gives me something to work with. Secondly, and more importantly, most of these people will be released at some point, and if I can stop them from reoffending by talking to them, I would be more than willing to talk to them as often as possible.

All people who are not mentally healthy are still human, and nearly everyone can be helped if we remember this fact. I'm not delusional, though, and I have looked into the eyes of some seriously evil people, both male and female. You see something very different between an individual who has harmed another, whether accidentally, in a moment of intense emotion, or as a result of mental illness, and a cold-blooded murderer. No one, or at least very few, thinks of themselves as "evil", and we can all find ways to justify our actions.

To summarise, mentally healthy people do not:

- Commit suicide
- Commit murder
- Commit rape
- Harass others in any way

Nor do they:

- Create false allegations
- Destroy a person's career over trivialities
- Spend time purposely looking for things to be offended by
- Blame anything but themselves for everything

I'll stop here because the bullet list could fill its own book. I may even write one. But, based purely on this short list, let me reiterate once more before going any further; no, it's not fucking "OK to Be Not OK". In a nutshell, what I want to cover in this work is that being "Not OK" is not OK, and normalising it as though it is OK and just how things are is causing more harm than good, both for the individual and humanity at large, especially when there is so much help available to feel OK! I'm also sick of the word OK already, so I will limit its use from here on in, OK? I shall instead refer to it as "the phrase".

3

Self-doubt is a Common Occurrence.

Have you ever had one of those days when it seems like a muse has whispered an inspirational idea in your ear out of the blue? You feel really good about the idea and are motivated to bring it to fruition. However, at some point before you've begun implementing the idea, self-doubt starts to creep in, and you wonder if the idea is genuinely any good or not. I assure you that you are not alone. If you wallow in it for too long, it will affect your mental health and prevent you from taking any action. If you then see your idea fully realised by another, this will only make you feel worse. I've experienced this so often, and it's slightly annoying to think how some of those ideas could have made me a fortune!

Not following your passions and realising life goals is a common cause for feelings of depression, and it is our anxieties which hold us back more than any external influence. I have wanted to share what forms the content of this book for several years, but I have been putting it off for various reasons. If I'm being brutally honest, one reason was I just couldn't be arsed to sit down and dedicate the time to write it all out, back it up with some facts, edit it and then go through all the hassle of trying to get people to read it. I'm past that now, having remembered that if you want to be what is often referred to as a "people helper", not only do you need to do the shit which will help them, but also elements which you don't enjoy. Writing and research are things I do enjoy. However, anything admin-related, as well as sales and marketing, is something I would definitely outsource if I could afford to do so. I know a fair amount about marketing, but I don't particularly enjoy it. I think the late comedian Bill Hicks made a lasting impression on me with his thoughts on marketers. If you want to know what he said, Google it, as it's not important to my point.

If I were to pinpoint the most significant reason for delaying my writing, it is this: the self-doubt that I may not know enough, I could be wrong in what I have to say, and I do not have the credibility to be taken seriously, a condition which you may have heard of called imposter syndrome. The condition itself is something I could write another book about, but not today. Today, I want to stick within the parameters of the book title with as few tangents as possible, but there will be some; I am well-known for them. For example, whilst I am not going to go deep into imposter syndrome, I want to share a little of my personal experience of it, so you can make an informed decision whether or not you think what I am sharing is credible or merely a load of shite. You may also be able to relate to parts of this story if you've experienced self-doubt based on your social class.

The first three years of my life were spent on or close to Army barracks, with the next seven years on council estates. I essentially left school with no qualifications and worked in a supermarket for a year before serving in the Royal Navy for nearly eight years. There are those in society who would describe someone with this kind of background as "working class scum". Not many would say it to your face, but I can assure you from experience that many think it and may mention the term when they don't realise the background of the person they are talking to. Whilst I don't see class as the determining factor of character or consciousness, this can't be said to be true for many people, whether this is looking down with disdain on a class lower than your own or looking up with a mixture of jealousy and hatred towards the higher ones. I mention this here because if you were born working-class, you would be aware of this kind of second-class status unconsciously, if not consciously, and it can contribute to a feeling of not being good enough when you try to follow your passions. It's something I've often struggled with.

In the book *A Dangerous Method* by John Kerr, which goes deep into the relationship between Sigmund Freud, Carl Jung and Sabina Spielrein, there is a reference to the working class being thought incapable of academic study at the time.[9] Unfortunately, I can't easily find this section of the book to use the actual quote because, unlike the movie version, which seems to focus mainly on Jung's fetishes, the book is based on letters, therefore factual, very wordy, and hard going even for those interested in the history of psychoanalysis.

This provides a nice segue into what I did after leaving the Royal Navy. Not many people leave the military to train in Hypnotherapy and Hypnoanalysis, certainly not many from the lower decks, but that's what I did in 1996. It was almost by accident, but that's another story and a tangent I shall not include here. That year marked the beginning of my interest, education, and research in human behaviour. I operated a small practice for three years but was not overly busy. For the next ten years, I worked part-time at a private health centre and achieved a success rate of over 90% with my clients. Most of the time, I felt confident in my abilities, not in a smug way, but more in the sense of "yeah, I've done something good today". I would then give it no further thought and switch from therapist mode to Navy Veteran mode and probably go for a few beers. Yet, those times I had not been able to help a client would stick in my mind.

I'd have thoughts such as:

- "I'm a fraud; I don't know what I'm doing."
- "I don't know enough. Should I be doing this?"
- "Am I merely a blagger?"
- "I should be able to help everyone, so what went wrong?"

Perfectionism and self-doubt are just a couple of the things you may experience with impostor syndrome. However, if you can look at the numbers detached from emotion, it makes no sense to feel like this if your successes heavily outweigh your failures. Any evidence that contradicts this negative self-view should be given serious consideration, as it demonstrates that the thought is invalid. Also, everyone struggles when starting something new; proficiency only comes from repeated practice.

That's enough of my impostor syndrome and working-class stigma; let's crack on with the main subject: mental health. I will not focus on the mental health issues I have faced too much, but I will mention personal experiences from time to time if I feel it could be helpful to do so. For example, I have struggled with depression intermittently for many years. Even though I generally think I'm over it, every once in a while, it can kick in and debilitate me for a day or two, usually with no apparent trigger. I did take medication for a while and visited some therapists and counsellors, but I mainly worked through it myself based on my knowledge and training. I mention this to assure you that I fully empathise if you feel this way.

It has also been pointed out by a couple of people that I seem to exhibit behaviours consistent with ADHD, so there's a possible third reason why it's taken me so long to get around to writing this book!

4

How Prevalent is Poor Mental Health?

If you want statistics, there's plenty to look at online, so I don't plan to get too carried away with them in this book, especially since I find compiling citations tedious. To cover my arse, I am providing references for anything which is not of my own creation in this book, whether I need to or not! You'll find them starting on page 127 if you want to verify anything.

It's virtually impossible to get an accurate idea of how widespread poor mental health is anyway, and as Homer Simpson points out, "Oh, people can come up with statistics to prove anything, Kent. 40% of all people know that".[10] However, I thought it would be helpful and, in some ways, comforting to look at the prevalence of mental health disorders in some of what are known as Western countries. I only say comforting so you know you are not alone. I apologise if I left your country out. You can quickly look up your country's stats using my data source. I also chose Western countries because I do not have enough experience or expertise to comment on improving the state of mental health in other regions of the world. While we may experience similar disorders, different cultures possess varied perspectives on life. As I previously stated, "horses for courses" and all that.

The upcoming four charts cover a period of thirty years. You may notice from the first two charts that the United States jumped significantly up the list of countries. You may be inclined to think this was due to the tragic events which occurred on September 11th 2001, in New York. However, this shift occurred in 1997, and although I tried to look online for a significant event which could account for this jump, I could not find one. I'm sure there must be one, and I'd be interested to know what it was. Other than this, the changes in rankings are relatively minor. I was more surprised to discover no fundamental changes in the figures in 2002, despite the "Global War on Terrorism" being in full swing by then.

The years were chosen arbitrarily because the most recent statistics from this source were for 2021. Therefore, I used this as my starting point, then went back ten years to compile my charts. I looked at each year individually when I did my research, but the increase has been gradual during this time frame. I could have shared many data charts I examined during my research, but I do not want to overwhelm you with information that does not provide any tangible benefit. Yes, it supports my claims, but it can also get really fucking boring, which tends to make people put a book down before finishing it. I am not writing this book to get a pat on the back from academics.

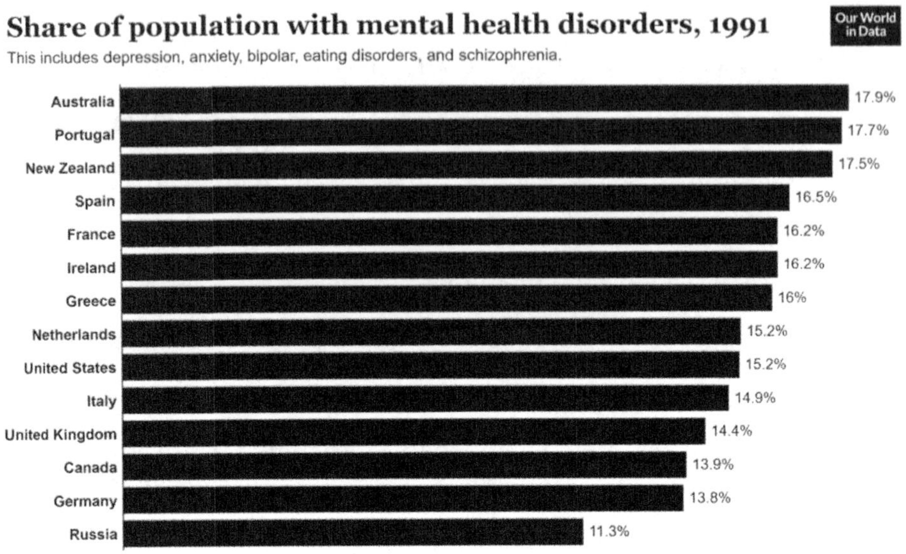

Chart 4 - 1991

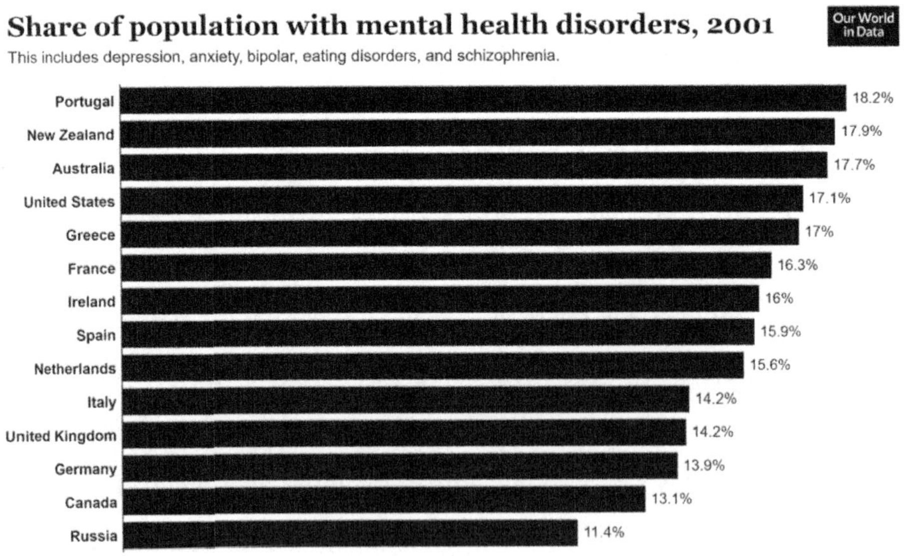

Chart 5 – 2001

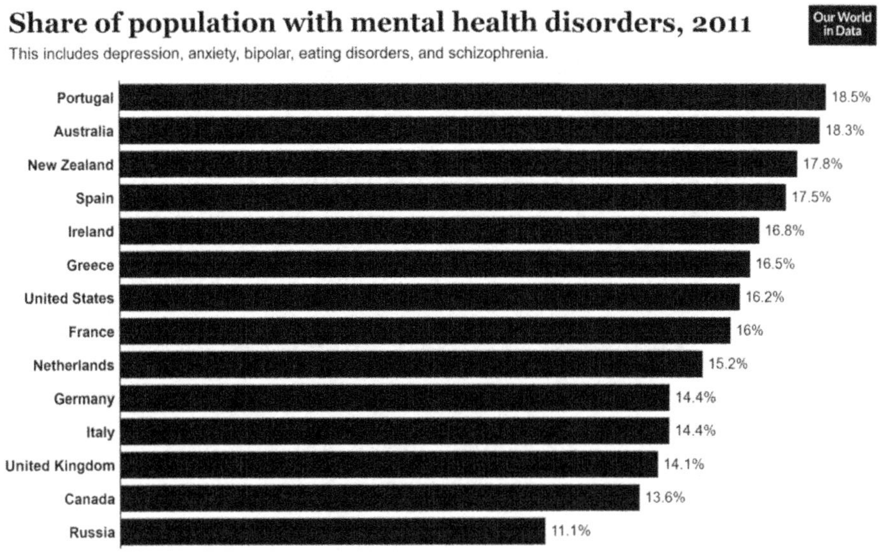

Chart 6 – 2011

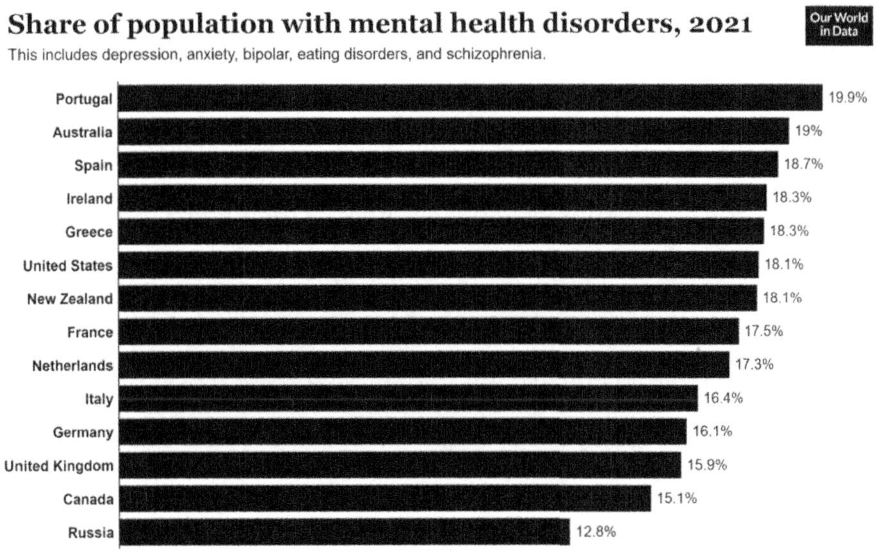

Chart 7 – 2021

Charts 4-7: IHME, Global Burden of Disease (2024) - with major processing by Our World in Data[11]

Many people blame social media for the rise in mental health issues; I have certainly been among them. I am still of the mind that it does play a factor, but maybe not to the extent I supposed. Looking at the ten years between 2001 and 2011 on the previous charts, we do not see a significant jump as expected if this were a major contributing factor. If we use Facebook as an example, it is still the most used platform at the time of writing, with 3.1 billion monthly active users. It was around 2006 when it started to become popular, and by 2008, it had over 100 million users. In 2011, monthly active users increased from 600 million in January to 800 million by September, according to Hootsuite.[12]

Despite legitimate complaints about social media platforms, such as spreading fake news, scams, clickbait marketing, and the rise of hate speech, they genuinely do not appear to have the significant overall impact we might have suspected. I will discuss social media and improving your mental health later in the book.

As I've already stated, I do not think we can get an accurate picture of how big a concern mental health is; more of a rough idea of the problem. This is because so many people suffer in silence. However, when researchers compile data like in the charts I've just shared, specific methods will be used consistently. So, if we look at most countries in the list, over the last thirty years, there has only been, at most, a 2% increase in mental health disorders. Don't get me wrong, this is still an increase of millions, but I'm hoping you see that although some make out as if it's a modern phenomenon, it has been a major concern for a very long time. We have neglected this matter for far too long, and it is finally time to give it the attention it deserves.

5

We're All a "Bunch of Balloons"!

In this day and age, there are many neurotics who get needlessly offended by words that quite often do not require offence. Even words generally accepted as offensive still depend on context and who is saying them. To illustrate, very few people complain when Samuel L. Jackson says a particular word, as he often does in movies. Whereas, if I were to say it publicly, there would be justifiable anger. You know the word I mean, and it's not "Mother Fucker"! You can say a sentence to one person who will laugh their cock off, but say it to another, and they'll kick your head in; it's context and setting, which is more important than the actual words used.

"Fake outrage" articles are showing up more and more in my timeline, and no matter how many times I click the three dots and select "not interested", "hide all", or "block", more of that type of shit still shows up. So, we must be careful when believing that certain things have upset a small minority of people when, in reality, they might not have. It's more likely to be some fucker fishing for likes or planting a divisive seed in your mind.

I've already pointed out the importance of humour and will try to inject some throughout this book. Yes, mental health is a serious subject, but we don't have to be solemn when we talk about it. I know some people will find some of my humour funny, and some won't. This is beyond my control, but I enjoy writing for those with a sense of humour rather than for the buzzkills. Depression and anxiety do not prevent a sense of humour; indeed, a sense of humour can sometimes alleviate the severity of both conditions. Yet, some seem to lack any sense of humour at all. I'm truly grateful not to be one of them.

The issue we will all face at some point in our lives is that what is deemed acceptable as a term today will inevitably become offensive in the future. Older generations are most likely to fall foul of these changes inadvertently, and not knowing is not considered a reasonable excuse. This issue has become increasingly prominent in the modern digital age, as numerous individuals seek to be outraged merely to attain their "fifteen minutes of fame" in the social media spotlight. One day, the word "water" could be offensive, and this book will be banned when that day comes. To be fair, it will no doubt be long before that because, besides what I know might upset some people, I am bound to have used a term unintentionally, which someone will be offended by. You would not believe how many seemingly innocent words I researched to see if they were already offensive to some. Pretty much every fruit and vegetable I looked up had a slang meaning or might upset certain people. The first non-offensive word I encountered was "water" on December 9, 2024, so this is what I chose to illustrate my point.

So, if some self-righteous shitbag reading this book decides to take offence at a word or phrase I've used, knowing full well it was not meant with that intent, then they are a total wanker and should go fuck themselves!

I was not being serious with that last sentence; I was merely giving an example to demonstrate what deliberately offensive looks like. I am very grateful that you are reading my book, and I want it to benefit you even if you get offended at any point. My whole intention in this book is to help whoever reads it. A very long-winded tangent there, albeit still relevant, so that I can explain this chapter's title.

When working in prisons, a term I often heard was "fucking balloon" when referring to someone's behaviour which was considered a bit stupid. There were a few cockneys where I worked, so if you hadn't guessed, it was a slang term for lunatic. Although this is not a term that I would use to describe anyone suffering from poor mental health, it can be used in jest between friends. Remember, context and setting are the most important factors. So, with this in mind, and in jest, the chapter title implies that we're all mad as a bunch of frogs. You can probably see why I felt it was important to share that lengthy tangent at the beginning of the chapter!

Seriously, though, I want to suggest that nearly everyone, if not everyone, suffers from poor mental health at some point, if not most of the time. In summary, I believe poor mental health boils down to anything we do which is destructive, whether that is a thought, the words we speak, or the actions we undertake. Passing this off as just being "human behaviour" should no longer be an acceptable excuse. Since most people do this daily in some way, even if it's only when they criticise or complain about something, I stand by this statement. I would imagine even the most devout spiritual practitioner has had doubts or a crisis of faith at some point, and this, too, could be considered to be having a poor mental health day. A better question, surely, is, "What is good mental health?"

According to the WHO, not the band but The World Health Organisation:

> Mental health is a state of mental well-being that enables people to cope with the stresses of life, realise their abilities, learn well and work well, and contribute to their community. It is an integral component of health and well-being that underpins our individual and collective abilities to make decisions, build relationships and shape the world we live in. Mental health is a basic human right. And it is crucial to personal, community and socio-economic development.
>
> Mental health is more than the absence of mental disorders. It exists on a complex continuum, which is experienced differently from one person to the next, with varying degrees of difficulty and distress and potentially very different social and clinical outcomes.[13]

The psychologist Abraham Maslow talked about self-actualisation in his work on the Hierarchy of Human Needs.[14] My favourite psychoanalytical author, Carl Jung, writes of self-realisation through individuation.[15] In psychotherapy, we also talk about a person becoming psychologically integrated, and there are many different approaches and theoretical perspectives to achieving this.

All that may have sounded like a load of psychobabble to you, and the internet is full of people using it. Some are students or practitioners of the subject, but nowadays, it's more common to see people using it to try to sound more intelligent than they are. Wherever possible, I try to put things in terms that anyone with a basic understanding of English can understand. That is the level of education I left school with, which I feel most comfortable with and use in most of my daily interactions.

So, to use words we can all understand, I think good mental health is the ability to react to what life throws at us with a level head and not let our emotions take control of our decision-making capabilities. By endeavouring to do this more often, we can become the best version of ourselves possible. I'm not suggesting you become an entirely logical and emotionless person like the Vulcans from *Star Trek*, but maybe not too far off from that level of personal control.[16]

A great way to start gaining control over your emotional state is to improve your ability to say "no" to requests from others when you don't want to do them. Additionally, it's crucial to develop the capacity to accept "no" when others decline your requests. Both of these skills can be more challenging than they seem. None of us likes to be turned down, but most people can quickly get over it. I firmly believe that the number of people unable to accept rejection in all its forms is increasing significantly; I will discuss this further in a later chapter.

We all have a darker side to our nature, called the shadow in Jungian psychotherapy. There is much more to it than this simple definition, but it will do for now. For the sake of this book, I want to draw your attention to just a couple of its negative aspects, although the Shadow also includes some positive facets. We all have thoughts that can be pretty disturbing when they come up, and we would never wish to tell others about them. These thoughts may be sexual in nature or involve harming yourself or others. Unless you are some sort of psychopath who would act upon them, when they come up, you should typically ask yourself, "Where the fuck did that come from?"

Another thing we do is project our unconscious weaknesses and negative behaviours onto others. In simple terms, you know that person who pisses you off when they act in a particular way? Well, maybe it's time you looked in the mirror to see how you behave that way, too. From my experience, the person exhibiting this bad habit usually does so in a more exaggerated way than we do it ourselves. I believe this is so that it highlights the behaviour more, like putting a giant neon sign above their head which reads, "You need to work on this shit!" For example, if someone irritates you for being extremely judgmental all the time, you might need to look at the times when you can be judgmental, too.

Working on your shadow is part of how you become the best version of yourself and involves repressed and denied behaviours specific to each individual. This is pretty advanced stuff, which isn't easy to do purely on your own without a trained professional, but you can make a start by simply admitting you have a shadow. The Shadow is not to be confused with the more universal instinctual behaviours we all have.

6

The Murderous Beast vs The Civilised Human

I'm keeping this ridiculously simple now and not putting forward a hypothesis for deep discussion. Plenty of people will bore you to death talking about the roles of different parts of the brain and use lots of technical terms associated with the mind, so I don't see the point in repeating any of it. It may well make yours truly appear to be superiorly intelligent, but it would be preposterously superfluous in a tome calculated to be understood by the simplest of intellects. Yes, I did write that last sentence as a piss-take, just for shits and giggles. It might not amuse you, but it made me laugh.

Anyway, for the sake of argument, let's say one part of us is instinctual and prioritises keeping us safe and getting our needs met. Given the right conditions, it is capable of destroying anything in its path using only its bare hands. This worked for your ancient ancestors; otherwise, you wouldn't be here to read these words. When something angers you, the Murderous Beast is ready to spring into action. A typical example: someone cuts you up whilst driving, and for a split second, you may feel that if you could get to that person, you'd rip their throat out with your teeth. What prevents you is the Civilised Human who thinks things through rationally and realises that although this event briefly endangered your life, it didn't actually cause you any harm, so it's OK to calm down. How long this takes varies from person to person and accounts for the differing responses we get, the worst cases being commonly known as road rage in this example.

A parent protecting their child from harm is likely to unleash the Beast quite quickly, and this would be a reasonable example of it doing its job in a justified way. We don't live in a utopia, and there are a lot of fucked up people on the planet. However, if the event happened when you were not there, the Beast being allowed to go out and seek retribution is not the appropriate response for a Civilised Human. We all know that revenge will not change the past, and depending on how it is carried out, it could end up with you being in prison for a long time. For many, this would be a price worth paying, and the ability to let go of the hatred will not be easy to achieve. I'm a Scorpio, and if you believe in such things, we're meant to be able to hold onto grudges for lifetimes. In the past, I can honestly say that I was indeed a typical Scorpio. These days, I like to think that regardless of the situation, if I were not present when it happened, I might initially contemplate my revenge, but ultimately refrain from acting upon it after careful consideration. On the other hand, if it happened in front of me, my control of the Beast may be limited.

The number of people who have wholly tamed the Beast and would not let it off its leash under any circumstances may be minimal, but they do exist. Here, I need to distinguish between two groups that fit into this description. The group I refer to is your Sages, Yogis and other Spiritually Enlightened individuals. Mohandas K. Gandhi is a good example of a person who employed this non-violent way of behaving.

Then, there are those who only unleash the Beast in their minds because their anxiety prevents them from taking any physical action; this is even worse for you. As neuroscience would confirm, being in this state for longer than necessary is not good for your physical health either. This heightened state of alert deactivates certain systems in your body and triggers the release of various chemicals. These chemicals evolved in us to help combat the real threats we faced daily throughout much of human history. If you're reading a book like this, I'm relatively sure you live in a reasonably safe environment compared to your ancestors.

At its core, this Murderous Beast focuses on just a few priorities: ensuring your safety, collecting and protecting its resources, and spreading its genetic material. It reacts when it fears that any of these things are in jeopardy. We see this late at night in pubs and clubs when the insecure male picks a fight because someone merely checked out his girlfriend. Mate, if she's heading home with you, you ought to be flattered that others view you as having an attractive partner.

Obviously, individuals are easier to manage than a pack of Murderous Beasts. We've all seen the often-comical videos of what happens when the doors open at department stores for various annual sales or the panic buying when an alleged shortage is announced; toilet rolls in 2020 spring to mind. But when this level of fear permeates a section of society, the Murderous Beast can be unleashed far too easily, where reason and common sense have little hope of intervening. History is full of many tragic and horrific examples of what happens when a mob get together, or a totalitarian government takes power. The masses can be swiftly divided and incited to turn against each other or target a specific small group in society. Often, this is by design and for various reasons, but primarily for the financial gain of a mere few. This is why it is imperative to be wary of any and all messages designed to elicit the emotions likely to unchain the Beast. Cunning manipulators craft these messages to exploit your anxieties and indignations. They are highly skilled at it, and most people will be taken in by it repeatedly, even after it has been pointed out. This, sadly, is the world we live in, but you can choose to be one of the people who doesn't participate or buy into this bullshit. I'm not putting a tin foil hat on and discussing conspiracy theories here. This shit goes on, and we all know it does. I choose to think of political propaganda more like a sport; you can actively participate or simply be entertained as a neutral spectator.

As a species, we do not appear to be learning from history, as advocates of the subject suggest we ought to. It has been over a century since Friedrich Nietzsche wrote, "In individuals, insanity is rare, but in groups, parties, nations, and epochs, it is the rule,".[17] We don't seem to be learning, do we?

We all have different personal triggers for what will unchain the Beast and to what extent it will be allowed to run free, but the less time it has, the better our physical and mental health will be. Some people claim they want to change the world for the better, but better how and for whom exactly? If they have to use their Beast to achieve it, is this truly a better world? If you ever go to a demonstration, rally or counter-demonstration, you will always find people on both sides eagerly awaiting the right catalyst to unleash the Beast.

If you want to make a difference in the world, the easiest thing to do is to start by developing your own Civilised Human. Anyone who thinks they can change everyone else in the world to suit their needs will find they have taken on an impossible mammoth endeavour. Either that, or they are barking mad!

7

"The Lunatics Have Taken Over the Asylum"

If you're into music, you will know this was the title of a song released in 1981 by Fun Boy Three, a short-lived band comprised of members of The Specials.[18] Although it could just as easily have been written today, the lyrics would be just as relevant. I take solace in the thought that even though society's problems haven't disappeared, I'm still here forty-three years later. However, what does concern me is that four decades ago, there was no internet, so although psychopaths may well have been in charge of many countries back then, too, your average everyday neurotic had little impact upon the rest of us with their personal opinions.

Back in the eighties, if you found a TV show offensive, you could write into the BBC's long-running *Points of View*, hosted by Barry Took and then Anne Robinson.[19] With only four TV channels at the time here in the UK, you would have caught at least a few episodes when there was nothing better on if you weren't an actual fan of the show. Having watched it with family as a child and later with friends, the general attitude when viewing an episode was to laugh at the absurdity of writing in and complaining.

This was usually followed by someone pointing out the obvious with one of three comments:

1. "What the fuck were you expecting to see in a film about…?"
2. "If you don't like it, don't watch it!"
3. "Hasn't this twat got something better to do?"

Nowadays, we have what has come to be known as "cancel culture", which in some instances may be warranted but, by and large, seems to be getting a bit out of hand. Context is ignored, and if you can amass enough likes on social media, anyone and anything can be brought down simply because one person doesn't like it. Plenty of supporters will rally to the cause if they think it makes them morally superior, even though they probably don't actually care.

As previously mentioned, what is "offensive" differs from one person to the next, and a healthy attitude is one where you can accept that you're not going to like everything someone does or says. Actively looking for something to take offence at is neurotic behaviour because what is essentially being said by such a person is, "The world should be how I want it," or "I can be me, but you shouldn't be you." With over 8 billion people on the planet, how narcissistic is this kind of attitude?

I feel the need to point out that, politically speaking, this way of thinking applies to both the left and right; only the specific "offences" differ. Whether this is due to some conspiracy of media design or not, I wouldn't like to say for sure, but I will say that it does not serve humanity. We've all heard the saying "divide and conquer." We can see people being divided over the most trivial things whenever we visit a social media platform.

I'll give a quick example of what I mean by trivial: any thread started on the subject of the post-George Lucas era *Star Wars* will have several types of comments:

- People who like the show/film
- People who do not like it for genuine individual reasons
- People who probably didn't watch it but want to complain about something they heard about it
- People who probably didn't watch it but want to say how innovative and refreshing it was
- People who spend a lot of time looking to call *Star Wars* fans names and accuse them of being bigoted, etc.[20]

The first two types are what you would expect from a healthy discussion from people with good mental health, whereas the others certainly fall into the category of neurotic behaviour. To date, I like most of what has been created in the *Star Wars* franchise, even though certain elements could have been done better for my liking. There are also a few additions to the franchise which I will never watch again. The great thing is that I have that option and do not have to watch them again, just as anyone who enjoys it can do so too. If I were to share online which bits I thought were shit, and why I thought so, undoubtedly, someone would be there instantly to comment with the standard insult of "fanboy". Is the irony of using this phrase not lost on them? Are they aware that there are Star Wars fans who are not male? Do they honestly think that I will change my mind by childish name-calling and suddenly like it? Or are they merely an antagonistic twat suffering from low self-esteem? I assure you, people with high self-esteem have far better things to do with their time.

If discussing trivial things in such an irrational manner, is it any wonder that the more serious, complicated and potentially sensitive societal issues are almost identical to forty years ago? The impersonal keyboard warrior approach to online communication has made adult discussion nearly impossible. With the chances of physical repercussions being slim, people have become emboldened to say things online they would never dare say to a person's face.

Virtue signalling manifests in various forms and is enacted by individuals across the spectrum of political and religious ideologies. If these individuals were as virtuous as they perceive themselves to be, surely the world would be a significantly better place. If someone is spewing hate towards the haters, judging the judgmental, and bullying the bullies, then they, by definition, embody these traits as well and possess no genuine moral superiority, only pomposity.

Extremely quick tangent: I recently read the word pomposity in a book, and it brought a smile to my face. This word needs to make a comeback to common usage. Let's see how many times I can use it again before the end of this book!

Society's problems do not disappear by banning or ignoring them, but through frank and open discussion. If people feel that their concerns are being ignored or that they are being condemned for them, they can easily be radicalised and then recruited by extremist groups. Most people are not at the extreme ends of the political spectrum and share more common ground than they realise. Few individuals who support the right are actually goosestepping fascists, just as those on the left are not all Marxists intent on seizing all your property, although clearly some are!

8

The Rise of Narcissism

Not all, of course, but many of today's so-called role models, leaders, and influencers are ego-driven narcissists. In other words, they do not give a fuck about you, only themselves. This is not exactly something new; only the number of people classed as authority figures has grown exponentially since the ability to share videos online has become extremely easy and ridiculously cheap. We all can exhibit egoism, meaning that we prioritise our wants and needs. However, when arrogance is involved, it often leads to a sense of entitlement and/or the tendency to condemn others or, at the very least, to dismiss their needs and desires. On the entitlement side of things, we've all read about bloggers and people on YouTube with a significant following expecting special treatment based solely on this credential, then acting like a spoilt child when told to fuck off.

Quite often, a person of influence is put on a pedestal by their followers; this is definitely not a good idea. All influential people have flaws, which can come as a disappointment when one is made public.

Actors, musicians, and sports personalities sometimes try to portray a squeaky-clean image when, in reality, they have a skeleton or two in the wardrobe. When this is the case, someone will reveal one at some point, either for money or revenge. In contrast, those with a bit of a rebellious or controversial personality can get away with quite a lot.

The narcissist will exploit particular groups of people by telling them exactly what they want to hear, which helps them to assume a higher position in society than they deserve. Although I want to avoid discussing politics in this book, I will give a recent poignant example from that world which illustrates what I am referring to. The person in question is no longer a politician, so what I am about to say is simply a historical analysis. All that follows is common knowledge and easily verifiable.

In 2016, the UK voted to leave the European Union in what came to be known as Brexit. If you are British, you can chill, please do not get triggered. I am not here to comment on whether this was a good idea or not; I am simply going to point out some very narcissistic behaviour that went on, which both sides of the argument became aware of over time.

Boris Johnson wrote two articles about the E.U., one for being a member and one against it. With ambitions of becoming Prime Minister, he published the latter and became a significant voice for the Leave campaign. Yet, on the day the result was announced, he looked visibly shocked and a little distressed at the outcome when first interviewed by reporters. Personally, I would put money on him actually voting to remain when he was in the booth, but that may just be me being cynical; we'll never know. Anyway, he clearly had no plan, so when David Cameron resigned, he didn't run for the Conservative Leadership position. Even when he eventually became Prime Minister, he still didn't have a plan but made all the right noises to keep his job. He managed to win by a landslide despite hiding in a fridge and avoiding real questions put to him by reporters in the run-up to a general election. He did this simply by repeating a couple of phrases, "Get Brexit Done" and "Oven Ready Deal". What the fuck this latter phrase meant, I have no idea, but people bought it. It just sounded like a lot of pomposity to me! It probably helped his case that the opposition leader had been constantly demonised by many of the UK's media outlets from day one in that role. However, in 2020, when the UK finally left the E.U., he had nothing left. The one banner he had to keep people following him was no longer there. He was high on a pedestal, and many eyes were focused purely on him now. Yes, there was the pandemic to contend with, and he was cut some slack for this initially. However, even his most ardent supporters began to turn their backs as scandal after scandal emerged, all of which he attempted to deny until the bitter end, no matter the evidence against him. This is all classic narcissistic behaviour. For the record, I am not against the man; he used to be an entertaining back-bencher. Being such a larger-than-life character, I think his ambitions were for a world that only exists in his head, and the actual responsibility he ended up with was too much. Unlike many politicians who rise to the top job, he was prominent in the public eye for many years before this. Based on what I saw of him, I think he probably did believe he could make Brexit an astounding success and become a true British hero loved by all the people. He probably didn't consider that it would still be such a highly divisive subject a decade later. He's fine, though; he makes more money now than he did as a politician.

Some people want to be a leader because of the power or fame they'll attain, some to spread a particular message, and some do it purely for the money. There's nothing wrong with making a lot of money if what a person does or shares is beneficial. Who wouldn't like to have a bank balance of millions? However, when that money goes to an individual's head, and they become supercilious, it might be wise to seek a new role model. OK, I've just got to throw in yet another tangent here, as I did say I like to use simple language that anyone can understand, and I just used the word "supercilious". Maybe you know what it means, but I admit I had never encountered it until about a year ago when listening to an audiobook. After looking it up in the dictionary, I thought, "What a great word, but when am I ever likely to use it?" As I typed the sentence, the word just automatically sprang to mind and at first, I thought I should change it to something else, possibly pompous. However, I may never get to use it again, so it's staying.

To clarify, this is the *Cambridge Dictionary* definition:

> Behaving as if you are better than other people, and that their opinions, beliefs, or ideas are not important.[21]

Anyway, back to my point. Do you think the world would be better if mentally healthy individuals, rather than those with fragile egos, were making the decisions? What a silly fucking question, right? Certain names may spring to your mind already, so that validates my point. However, you may think I'm just talking about decision-makers globally or nationally, but I also mean the narcissists that saturate all levels of society, from education to the workplace. While I won't share any here, during my research, I observed many bizarre policies implemented by managers who clearly wanted to be seen as "doing something" regardless of reason or practicality. Inclusivity should be commended, as nobody should feel they are being shut out based on personal characteristics. Still, policies must be fully contemplated to be sure they don't have the opposite effect. Sadly, this seems to be happening more and more to the detriment of humanity's evolution. I think there's more anger being generated by some ideas than actual benefits, but that may have been the plan all along. There's more profit to be made when people are divided rather than united.

When we have good mental health, it's easier to spot the limelight narcissist and not be fooled by their rhetoric. Getting people the right help at the right time is one of the antidotes to this rise of narcissistic behaviour. Since I think everyone suffers from poor mental health, we need to be working on getting rid of the remaining stigma surrounding the subject.

9
Mental Health Stigma

Every May is designated as Mental Health Awareness Week, and in some countries, the observance extends throughout the entire month. Its origins date back to the 1940s and 1950s, but it became such a well-known event only with the rise of social media. So, whilst I'm not a fan of most social media platforms in general, I have to concede that they do some good, too.

In addition to the above, every 10th of October is World Mental Health Day. During these times, social media will be swamped by savvy marketers making offers or sharing articles to capitalise on mental health's moment in the spotlight. I've never done this, and I do not plan to, as it feels to me like a bit of exploitation of the vulnerable. I find this to be especially true when the writer of the article, or the product being sold, has nothing to do in any way, shape, or form with treating mental health. For example, I created a website many years ago for Veterans diagnosed with PTSD, which was primarily to promote my book, but also has various support links on it. Any military-supporting charity or not-for-profit organisation can have a free ad on the website. However, I often receive emails, primarily from America, from companies that sell various items, such as mattresses, inquiring whether I would put a link to their website on mine for free, merely because they have an article about PTSD. My policy for accepting this type of link is that the advertiser must purchase a copy of my book, as my share of the profits goes to a military charity. This would demonstrate sincerity towards veterans' concerns. The book costs less than the price of three pints of beer down at the local pub. They can always donate the book if they don't want to keep it. I don't think this is too much to ask, do you? To date, only one of these enquiries has resulted in an ad being posted!

A better illustration of this disingenuous behaviour would be the number of companies donning rainbows on their products during Gay Pride month to garner more profit whilst doing very little or diddly-squat to help the LGBTQ+ community. I know that some big companies do a great deal for this community and donate to charities. However, there are others who, in my mind, hypocritically make donations to the cause whilst also contributing to the campaign funds of anti-LGBTQ+ politicians. Some don't even do that; they just reap the benefits of the rainbow. The same could be said for the Remembrance Poppy, too.

In other words, some advertisers lack integrity during big "official" days, weeks or months. I mention this because while publicly, they want to be seen doing some "good", they probably do not actually care, so the stigma still exists in their day-to-day business dealings. It's something to be aware of, especially before parting with money.

For the record, I'm not gay, but I do believe that it is entirely up to consenting adults to decide how they get their sexual kicks and nobody else. Let's face it: everyone is a cocksucker and/or a muff diver, a giver and/or a taker; if not, then they're probably just a wanker!

Anyway, with that tangent out of the way, let's proceed. There has been significant progress in reducing stigma for those suffering from mental health issues. Generally speaking, it is no longer considered a moral failing or sign of weakness, as the Ancient Greeks believed, and in the Western World, very few consider it a sign of possession by the Devil. However, there are certainly congregations in the U.S. who would disagree. The asylums of the Victorian age may be long gone, but a large proportion of society still shuns those with more severe personality disorders. We are slowly making progress in the right direction. However, people born with permanent conditions will experience stigma more than those who are only experiencing a temporary, treatable condition.

During my research, I read an article from the National Library of Medicine, which does seem to support my observation:

> The societal and individual effects of stigma are broad and pervasive. Stigma translates into individual reluctance to seek care, mental health professional shortages, and societal unwillingness to invest resources into the mental health sector. Yet, the research, teaching, and programming resources targeted to redress prejudice and discrimination remain a low priority, small in scale, and individually focused. With indications that the level of stigma may be reducing,

> strategies to identify factors associated with the decrease in stigma for depression, to address stagnation or regression in other disorders, and to reach beyond current scientific limits are essential to confront mental illness's contribution to the global burden of disease and improve population health.[22]

Things have come a long way in just my short time working with mental health. When I was first in practice back in 1996, people mainly suffered in silence from some of the common anxiety and depression disorders. Asking a client to recommend me to a friend who might benefit from my support nearly always resulted in a look which I translated to mean, "My friends have no idea about my condition, and I like it that way." By the late 2000s, though, with the advent of social media and people beginning to share "everything" online, clients would openly offer to promote me to their friends and family.

Fast forward to today, and every social media platform which lets you share videos is full of people talking about the state of their mental health. I would say some are genuine, and others may not be suffering as much as they claim. People facing more serious conditions now endure months of waiting just for a diagnosis, delaying their access to treatment that could help them maintain a more stable life.

A single mother recently shared that she might wait as long as eighteen months for an appointment with a specialist to address her belief that her six-year-old son has ADHD.

Much like the waiting times at A&E departments, this delay could be significantly reduced if individuals with easily treatable at-home conditions got out of the queue.

10

Hypochondria & Self-diagnosis

What follows is not to belittle anyone, especially anyone genuinely suffering from an anxiety disorder. Still, it is something that needs to be said, and as no one else seems to have the balls to say it, I shall. Everyone experiences anxiety from time to time. There is a significant difference between manageable fear and severe conditions like PTSD or phobias. Just saying you have anxiety doesn't mean you have a diagnosable anxiety condition; there may be other things going on, or maybe nothing. The best way to ensure accuracy is to consult a professional; however, it is essential to first determine if it is merely a natural off-day. Many assume they have an issue after conducting a Google or social media search. When we do this, we nearly always imagine a worst-case scenario.

As I mentioned earlier, the first recorded use of "the phrase" appears to have surfaced online in 2013. This was shortly before I began to notice behaviours I hadn't seen before. Specifically, people expressed that they were experiencing poor mental health, accompanied by statements that included the words "my anxiety." The behaviour which I found odd was that when mentioning “my anxiety”, it was being said with what I can only describe as pride, almost like a badge of honour, as if they felt special, even superior, for feeling anxious. They may also use anxiety as an excuse to avoid taking action themselves or, more commonly, to attempt to change someone else's behaviour. I observed these occurrences in both strangers and people I knew. I will share a couple of examples, though I could easily provide many more.

Example 1 – Total Strangers

Whilst it can be hard to get me to shut up once I start talking, especially if beer has been involved, I generally prefer to sit back and listen to others. You learn much more by listening, and this quote attributed to Plato sums this idea up succinctly: “Wise men speak because they have something to say; Fools speak because they have to say something”. Apparently, there is no record of this appearing in his writings. Damn you, internet, for making me believe it was an actual quote for so long! So sorry, Plato, no citation for you, sir. Tangent over.

So, there I was, sometime between 2016 and 2019, working as an actor on a low-budget short film, using a local pub as the set. Three of us formed the main cast, accompanied by about twenty extras and the crew, totalling roughly fifty people in a relatively small space. We were there for five days, so as an actor, there was a lot of downtime between camera set-ups. Some of this time would be spent running lines for the next scene, but I spent more time sitting and listening to what was happening.

By the second day, two crew members from the props and wardrobe department had caught my attention, and for the next couple of days, I listened intently to what they had to say, which revolved around a single topic: their anxiety. It was pretty much the same conversation, but retold to a different person each time. I'm reasonably sure everyone on set got the opportunity to listen to it, but I heard it many times while sitting in the background. Both talked about having social anxiety to start with, before getting into what can only be described as a competition about who had it the worst by providing examples of previous anxiety attacks. They both displayed confident body language when recalling one of these alleged events. They were smiling as they spoke, occasionally laughing, but not in a nervous kind of way. While I didn't directly ask any of the following questions, they did occur to me. In a therapeutic setting, I would have certainly asked some of them.

"Considering that you are in a relatively small space with many unfamiliar people and some from your peer group:

- Are you not afraid of being judged for sharing this very personal information?
- You seem very relaxed and calm; is this how you genuinely feel currently, or is it a front you are putting on?
- For a person suffering from social anxiety, you don't seem to have any problem starting a conversation with strangers on this film shoot. Is there a reason you feel able to do this?
- When reliving one of your experiences of an anxiety attack, can you explain why you show no physical signs of emotion?"

The last question is a bit of a dick question, for sure, because I'd be calling them out for being full of shit. It's not a question I would probably ask in a client session unless it was to elicit a particular response, which I believed could give them a breakthrough. But it's still something I would love to have asked in this instance to see their response. This is known as *Provocative Therapy*, which was devised by Frank Farrelly and is something I only ever used sparingly when in practice.[23]

As it was, I didn't ask any of these questions but instead interrupted one of these retellings with, "Before I got into acting, I worked as a psychotherapist for thirteen years. Have you looked into getting any help with your anxiety?" or words to that effect. I also mentioned I'd written a book for Veterans suffering from PTSD. Strangely, this was the first time I saw a single anxious physiological response in either person. It was almost like the proverbial rabbit in the headlights. They froze for about ten seconds and then looked at each other briefly before returning to the conversation without missing another beat, behaving as if I had not spoken at all.

During what was quite possibly a midlife crisis, where I trained and worked as an actor and filmmaker, I saw this kind of thing more times than I can remember now, but this was the most extreme version. Most other times, when I revealed my therapy credentials, I was not wholly ignored, and a conversation would ensue. I also spoke with people who genuinely had anxiety disorders and offered some advice or support.

Example 2 - People I Know Very Well

Even though I am a trained and experienced therapist, when it comes to close connections, I can still miss signs of poor mental health, and people can be very good at hiding what's going on internally. As I don't currently offer therapeutic services, I only tend to switch into therapist mode when someone comes to me with a problem. They may not always ask for this input, but they'll usually get it anyway.

My analysis in this example could be off, but I'm reasonably confident. This illustration involves two people who are related and roughly of the same age. One of them has suffered from panic attacks on and off for a couple of decades. The other has rarely shown any level of apprehension in any situation and is very confident, bordering on cocky twat. Don't get me wrong, the latter does have issues, but I have never seen a single indicator of anxiety. I did a couple of sessions with the former many years ago, but could not go as deep as needed for the numerous reasons that exist when working with a friend or relative. I have also talked with them over the telephone to help them overcome panic attacks. Even still, I have seen other occasions where they have used their condition to avoid stuff they didn't fancy doing. But hey, that's one of the perks of having a genuine condition; you can sometimes use it to your advantage. Most people won't know, but there are subtle signs you can't easily fake. Secondary benefit syndrome is one of the many ways people gain from having a condition. It almost reflects a common aspect of human nature: some individuals will take advantage of any systems put in place designed to help. The only difference is whether it is done consciously or not.

As for the other person, I overheard them arguing with another family member, and they were not winning. As a last-ditch attempt to get their way, they threw their ace in the hole, "Shut up, you're triggering my anxiety". Surprise, surprise, they then got their way.

While anxiety conditions are indeed on the rise, I've also noticed many instances of people faking these conditions for attention or to manipulate situations. This behaviour seems to be quite widespread. I'm not passing judgment on these individuals, who may well need therapy and might actually have low levels of anxiety. However, due to long wait times for professional consultations, I would prefer to see severe cases addressed more quickly. This won't occur as long as some individuals are motivated by the advantages of being perceived as a victim. A book I am writing in tandem with this one goes deeper into these benefits, so be assured I am not making this up.

So, how big a problem is anxiety, really? That's a great question! I'm pleased you asked, as I do have some data on the prevalence of anxiety disorders to share on the following pages, but not too much.

11
How Common Are Anxiety Disorders?

According to the World Health Organisation:

> An estimated 4% of the global population currently experience an anxiety disorder. In 2019, 301 million people in the world had an anxiety disorder, making anxiety disorders the most common of all mental disorders.[24] Although highly effective treatments for anxiety disorders exist, only about 1 in 4 people in need (27.6%) receive any treatment. Barriers to care include lack of awareness that this is a treatable health condition, lack of investment in mental health services, lack of trained health care providers, and social stigma.[25]

There is debate over whether PTSD is still considered an anxiety disorder. The UK's NHS believes it is, and that works for me.[26] This is how I referred to the condition in the book I wrote in 2011 for Veterans suffering from it. Seeing as PTSD was not included on the page the above quote from the WHO was taken from, it's worth considering that the global figure would be much higher than 4% if it were. Due to the numerous ongoing conflicts across the globe, the number of individuals experiencing the traumas of war, such as combat troops and the increasing number of civilian refugees caught in these situations, likely reaches the tens of millions.

As you'll see shortly in the last eight charts I'm going to share, age doesn't appear to be a significant contributing factor when it comes to anxiety disorders. The first two charts are to give a global overview. The following two are for the UK, because that's where I live, followed by two for Europe as a whole, and finally two for the USA. Once again, I'm using 1991 and 2021 for the three-decade comparison. Anxiety levels begin to spike in people in the Western world around the time they hit puberty. This shouldn't surprise anyone who has teenage kids or remembers what it was like when they were one. In the UK and Europe, numbers drop slightly after reaching young adulthood. In the United States, levels appear to continue to rise until reaching the mid-forties. Overall, there hasn't been that much change globally over the last thirty years. We don't see as significant an increase as you might imagine over the three decades, and the charts look almost identical in their age breakdowns. The most considerable increase appears to be in those under thirty. I do not think we can point fingers at a single cause for what is causing an increase in anxiety in the younger generations. However, I do suggest it is essential that we spend more time and money on research rather than knee-jerk reactions.

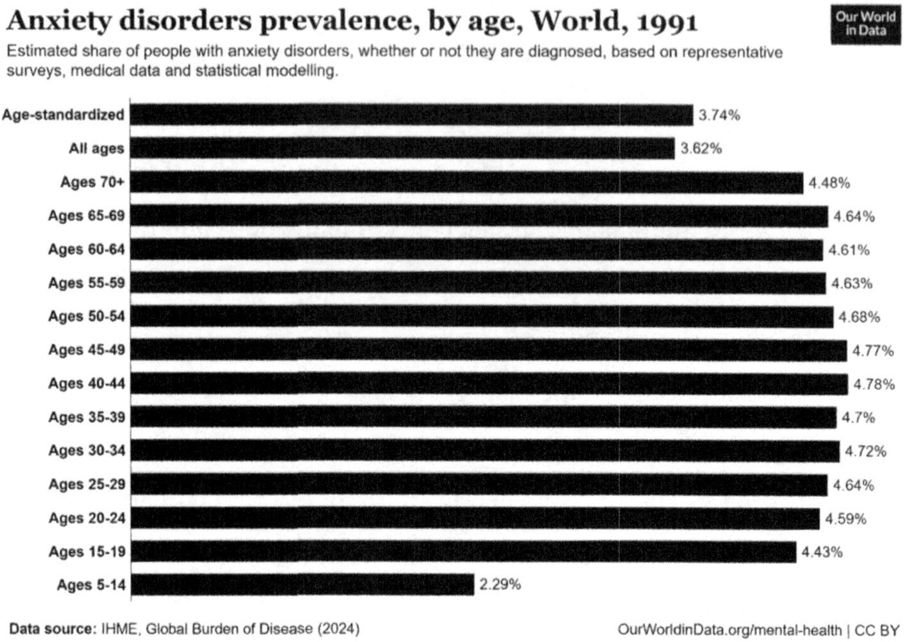

Chart 8 – World 1991

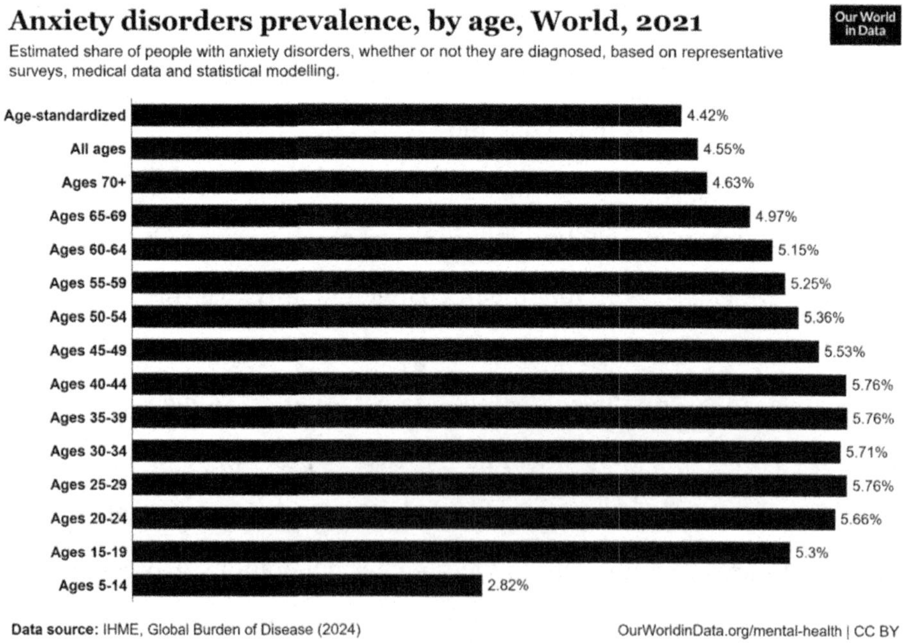

Chart 9 – World 2021

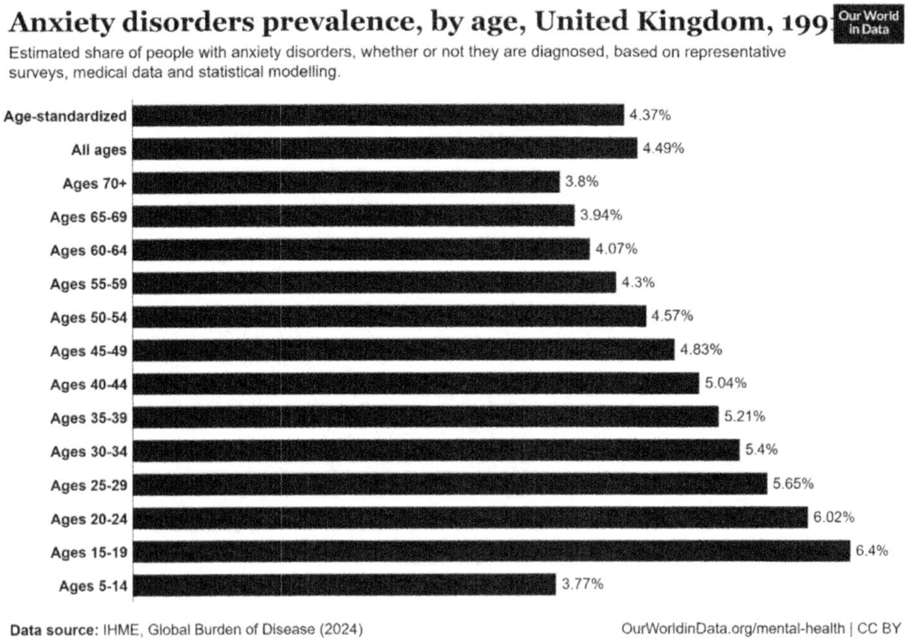

Chart 10 – UK 1991

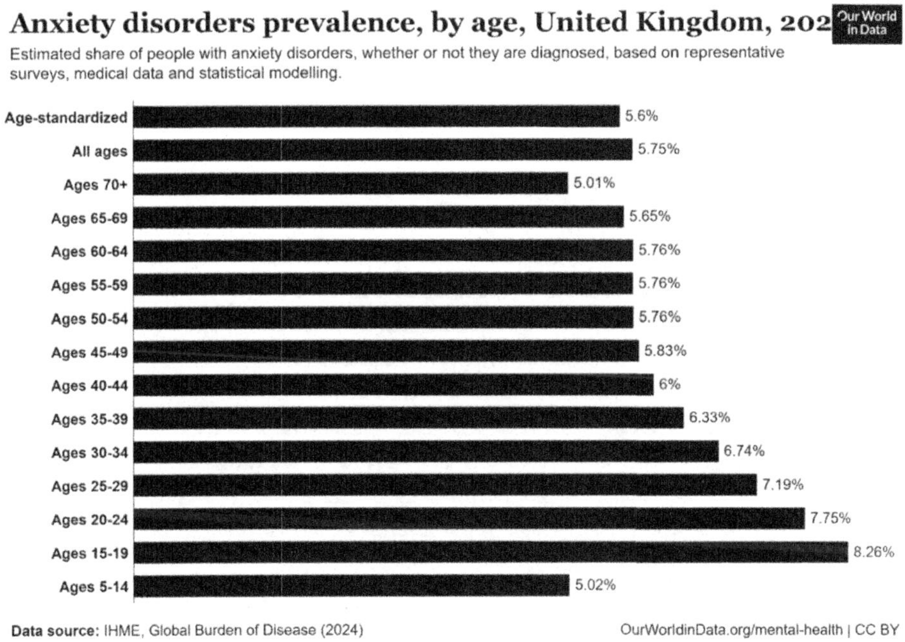

Chart 11 – UK 2021

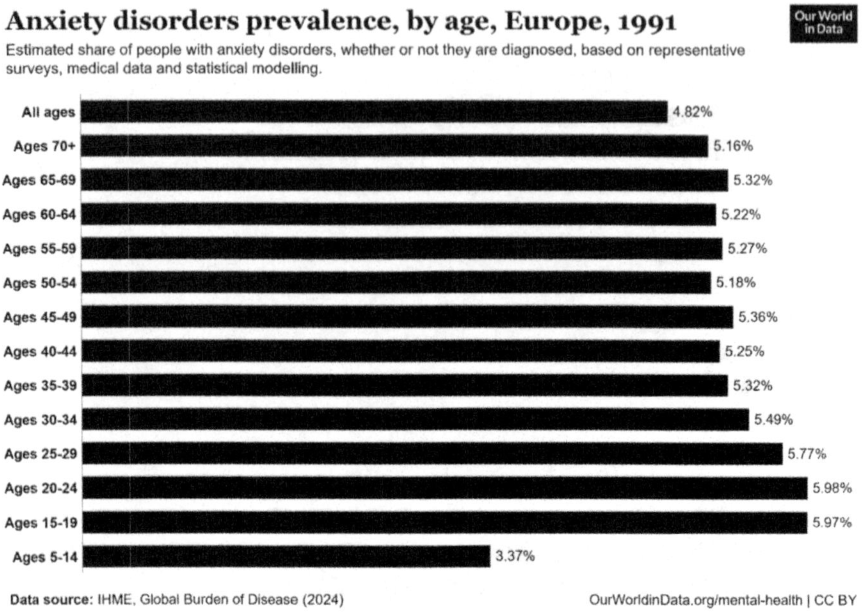

Chart 12 – Europe 1991

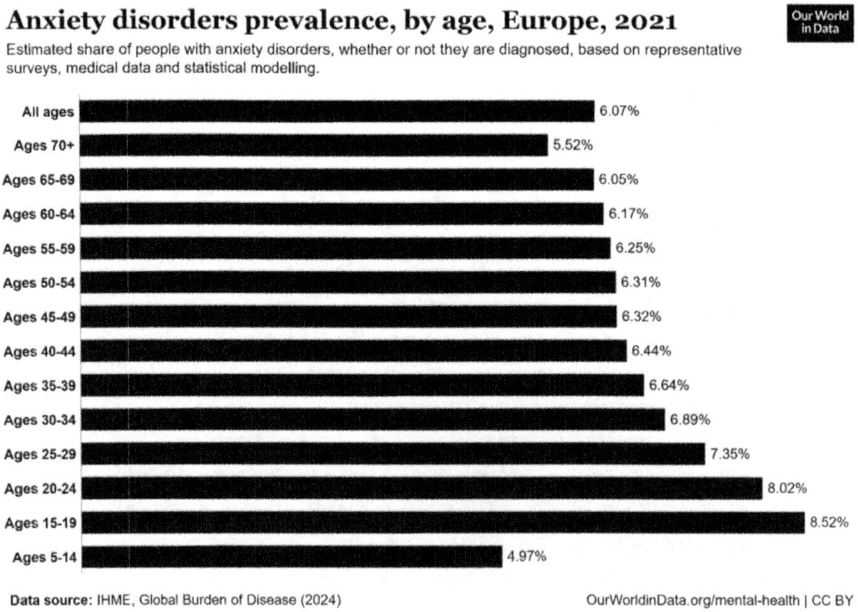

Chart 13 – Europe 2021

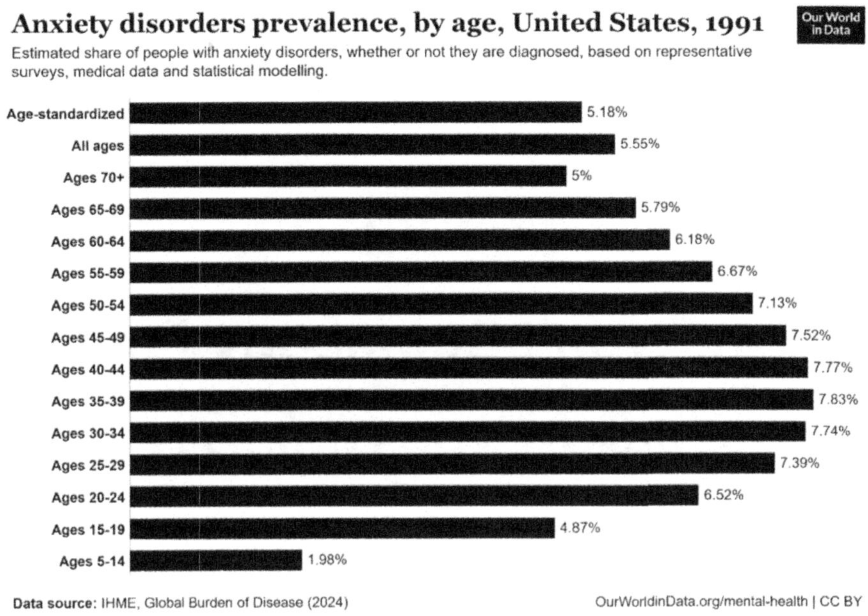

Chart 14 – USA 1991

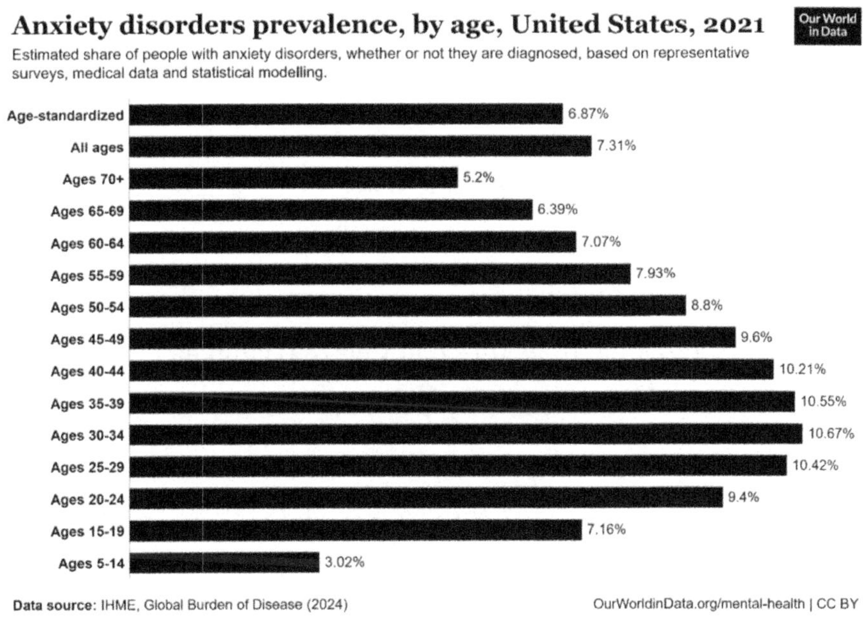

Chart 15 – USA 2021

Charts 8-15 IHME, Global Burden of Disease (2024) – with major processing by Our World in Data[27]

12

"Oh, Won't Somebody Please Think of The Children?"

OK, I couldn't help myself there; I had to throw in another Simpsons quote, this one being from Helen Lovejoy.[28] I thought it would be a good idea to take a brief comical pause because, in a moment, I will talk about my biggest concern with "the phrase" and how it relates to children. Now might be a good time to get up and stretch your legs and maybe put the kettle on before we continue.

During my research, I saw different figures relating to the increase in anxiety disorders in children, with some saying there has been as much as a 29% increase in a year. By now, you should know my thoughts on statistics in this area. The previous charts would seem to disprove what was likely a sensationalist article, as this increase appears to have taken thirty years. The numbers are irrelevant; one child suffering from anxiety is one too many.

I'm not a parent, but I do know many people who are. I've worked with children as an entertainer, whilst the parents use the couple of hours of respite to gossip amongst themselves. I also have parents. From listening to parents in various settings, I gather that many believe they are experts on raising children, and if you haven't got any, your opinion does not count. Bollocks to that; I've seen far too many examples of what can result from bad parenting to buy into any of that pomposity and bullshit.

I believe, similar to my views on therapy, that there is no single way to raise a child; it's more of an approach akin to "horses for courses." This said, I believe that parents universally have two essential responsibilities. We can see both of these duties in much of the animal kingdom. The first is obvious and one which most parents do naturally; they will prioritise their child's safety, even at the cost of their own lives. The second is not so easy, and I think it is a contributing factor to why we are seeing the rise in poor mental health among children, that of preparing them for adulthood and the perils that await them.

In my opinion, we overemphasise attention to the first role while neglecting the second. I've seen way too many times the negative repercussions of the overly protective parent who essentially wraps their child in cotton wool long into their teenage years. Insufficient preparation can leave individuals lacking the social and life skills to navigate life's challenges, leading some adults to retreat and stay in their "safe zone."

When I say preparing them for adulthood, I do not mean moulding them into what a parent thinks they should be. For example, if a parent wanted to be great at a particular task but never achieved it, they then try to use their child to compensate for this failure. If a child has a natural talent, that is different and should be encouraged.

When animals and birds reach a certain point in their development, their parents step back and only assist when necessary. They will have taught their offspring, through example, how to acquire sustenance, hide from predators, and defend themselves. As humans, we have to develop many more skills on top of these, and striving to get the right balance between protection and preparation is no easy task.

As I mentioned earlier, developing firm psychological boundaries involves being able to say “no” and hear it from others. I am not one of those who stereotype entire groups as "all being the same." This also applies to generations. There may be some reasonably common traits due to the various influences of the time you are raised, but not to the extent that it defines an entire age group.

For example, a person born at the start of the 20th Century would be very accustomed to hearing no. Whereas, the latest generation appears to struggle with not getting their way. Could this be down to participation trophies rather than healthy competition with clear winners? Is giving children a screen to look at rather than an experience of the outdoors contributing to this increase in self-centeredness? When parents concentrate their social time almost exclusively on their children, does this hinder the natural process of maturation and development? I am inclined to believe they have certainly contributed to the significant rise in this behaviour, but self-importance is not a new phenomenon.

Wanting the best for your children is only to be expected, as is not wanting them to go through the crap you did. If only a perfect guide existed for parenting that addressed every possible scenario. Unfortunately, there isn't one. Instead, we have the "experts" who promote their own method and parents who imitate or act contrary to their own.

Opinions are indeed divided on the various ways people will "swear by" what is the right or wrong way to raise a child. How to chastise a child who is playing up is probably one of the most contentious subjects. It's not a debate I intend to try to settle either. Where to place the line between what is discipline and what is cruelty generally falls into one of three camps. Some would never physically reprimand a child under any circumstances. Others think it is fine as long as it is done as a last resort and never excessively, and then others think it teaches respect because "It never did me any harm, and I turned out all right, didn't I!" To the latter group, I have to ask the question, "How do you know?" There is no way to compare how you would have turned out if raised differently.

As a child, I recall experiencing a sense of fear at times more than I now believe was necessary. I certainly wasn't abused by the standards of the day, and overall, I think I had a reasonably happy childhood. However, this fear undermined my confidence in many areas, some of which I didn't overcome until my late teens/early twenties and a few that are still not fully resolved but do not affect my day-to-day life. If I had been raised differently, who knows what a more confident version of myself would have become? Recalling what I was like as a teenager, I'd probably have fallen in with the wrong crowd and either be in prison or dead, but there's no way to know.

Would I still have dedicated years of study to human behaviour? Would I still have trained to become a therapist? Would I still be writing a book like this? Maybe I needed to go through some shit to be able to talk about it. Perhaps I was born to be a writer, no matter what, or maybe it's a little bit of both. This brings up another contentious debate on human behaviour.

13

Nature vs Nurture

Here again, we have three basic philosophies: those who think you're born one way and that's just how you are, those who think you can mould a child into anything you want, and those of us who think it's a little bit of column A and a little bit of column B.

In the works of the late Professor David R. Hawkins, a medical practitioner and psychiatrist, he suggests we are all born at a certain consciousness level. If you'd like to learn more, the most famous of his books is Power vs Force.[29] I find his books fascinating, and he has been an influence on my own work. I won't go deep into my theories about consciousness in this book; that'll be one further down the line. Suffice it to say, these levels theoretically account for why some children get pleasure from helping others while others like to be cruel.

Did you ever go to school with someone you'd describe as a "little shit"? If you are still aware of them, did they turn out to be a bit of a wanker as an adult? Did you ever know someone who was given everything they ever wanted and still acted like a spoiled brat? Did they turn out to be an adult twat too? You could say this is the "nature" part of the equation.

I can't speak about recent times, but there was always at least one school bully in my day. Some would be the popular children and the "jocks," as Americans tend to call them. There would also be one or more of these bullies that would come from the local "family", which would be pretty large and literally thick as thieves. Like a poorer version of the mafia, this family would be well known and maybe feared by any locals who knew them, as they had the numbers on their side. Multiple generations would carry on the family tradition, with plenty of lackeys to help them out. If something dodgy happened, their name would be the first to be associated with it. However, there would be a couple of members who didn't naturally fit the family mould. One might be the polar opposite of what was expected and never be involved with day-to-day business. Another might toe the line, but wasn't a perfect fit. They'd be the ones who seemed quite normal when none of the family was around; in other words, they were being "nurtured" to grow up a certain way. If we think of one of the most famous Mafia-related movies, *The Godfather*, there are the three Corleone brothers, Sonny, Michael, and Fredo.[30] Sonny was "naturally" a fit for the family business, but Michael was "nurtured" into it by circumstances, even though neither he nor his father wanted it to turn out this way. As for Fredo, he was kind of the runt of the litter. We may not be able to change the nature part easily, but according to many consciousness experts, it is certainly doable. On the other hand, we can definitely work on the nurturing part.

14

Hugs Not Drugs

A phrase from the eighties which had little to no impact on illegal drug use, but I'm stealing it for better purposes. I'm not talking about the fun type of drugs or even the ones which we associate with addiction and ruining lives. I know some will say they all ruin lives. Statistics show they don't "all" ruin lives, but I'm not going to share any here other than the fact that alcohol is the most destructive of drugs, and it's totally legal. As an ex-sailor, I can live with that. The late comedian Bill Hicks does a great routine on the subject of recreational drugs, which you can easily find online, and I highly recommend a watch. While this may oversimplify the issue, the risks linked to drug use often arise when someone lacks experience or turns to substances to avoid the realities of everyday life. But as I said, these are not the drugs I wish to discuss.

No, when I say "Hugs, not Drugs", I'm talking about the ones which are being given to children legally. Yes, some conditions require ongoing medication, but for others, they are being used far too soon and far too frequently for my liking. I am no doctor, so let me make this clear: I am not advising anyone to stop or refuse prescribed medication. When I chose to quit the medication that I had been prescribed for depression, it was only after having a consultation with my GP, who had been seeing me for over a decade. He only agreed to this because he was aware of my training as a therapist, and I explained how I planned to manage my condition. However, I do think parents should be more aware than they generally are about potential side effects and effectiveness. I am not alone; far better-qualified people have their concerns, too.

The following is an excerpt from an editorial published in Frontier Psychiatry:

> The accessibility and acceptance of a biological psychiatry treatment model have contributed to poorly evidenced treatments becoming common for paediatric mental health services. Most concerning is the fact that the number of youths receiving antipsychotics has increased by 50%-200% over the past 20 years, depending on the cohort. Further, most of the antipsychotic use in youth targets non-psychotic conditions and have not received approved or licensed labelling, thus, is 'off-label' or unapproved. Polypharmacy, i.e. combining classes of psychotropics, despite the lack of robust evidence that benefits outweigh risks, has also sharply increased. As with antipsychotics for behavioural use, 3-class polypharmacy lacks evidence that benefits outweigh risks. Unfortunately, parents are

> seldom aware of the risks (e.g. weight gain, metabolic changes, diabetes, sedation, tremor, somnolence, and restlessness) associated with these medications and, at times, are not fully engaged in the decisions to use them. The effects of polypharmacy are largely unstudied, and there are significant concerns about drug interactions.[31]

That quote might take a few readings to get your head around, and if you choose to read the full article, I assure you it doesn't get any easier. However, if you have a child currently on medication, I would advise you to have a look at it. Being better prepared will help you to ask the right questions when you speak with your doctor.

This excerpt from an article published in the British Medical Journal should be easier to digest:

> Many drugs given to children in the United Kingdom are unlicensed or prescribed "off-label." The so-called off-label prescribing of a licensed medication to a patient outside the specification of the product licence involves medicines being administered by an unlicensed route, in an unlicensed formulation or dosage, or to a child below the stated age range.[32]

In my view, this suggests that parents should focus on offering more emotional support and teaching children resilience before considering the use of drugs. If these drugs are designed for adults, it seems to me that only adults should be taking them, at least until the proper studies have been carried out. Instead, we should prioritise looking to reduce as many of the causes of poor mental health in children as possible. At the same time, we need to help them develop confidence, flexibility, and compassion.

Something to consider: every individual society and history has labelled as evil was once a child. Some may have turned out this way due to nature, but I'm sure some would have turned out differently with better nurturing. Young children are highly impressionable, and parents are usually the first port of call when they look for examples to imitate. I think it's vitally important that, for the child's sake, a parent should exhibit the right behaviours both online and in the real world. Parents tell children not to call people names, not to sulk, and not to mimic what everybody else is doing, plus many other things the child then sees the parent do. This likely contributes to their rebellion against their parents' preferences and the values they believe that generation stands for. Adolescents and young adults believe they will be the ones to improve the world and think they'll be different when they become parents themselves. Ironically, most people still turn out to be like their parents when they get to this point, with maybe a few subtle differences.

If you are under thirty-five and not yet a parent, consider this: you know that boring twat mowing his lawn who doesn't get it and says things which you find offensive; whom you may refer to as "boomer"? Well, they probably weren't like that when they were your age or younger. The "Baby Boomers" were born between 1946 and 1964. This means they were the original rebellious generation: the Teddy Boys, the

Mods and the Rockers, and the Punks who often got into trouble and thought their parents were "square". They were the hippies dropping LSD and smoking weed. They were the ones marching for peace and civil rights. Now look at them; this will likely happen to you, too! For the record, I'm mid-generation X, and we went to illegal raves, got absolutely spangled, and most of us did not give a fuck about a person's skin colour or sexuality. We were also a big part of the Goth and Indie scene. Let's see if you can beat all these older generations' achievements; as the saying goes, "I'll wait!"

Now that we're coming to the end of this chapter, I felt the need to bring back a little of my humour. It's tough being a parent, so I will cut them some slack and point out that their influence on their children reduces significantly and switches to friends and acquaintances as they age. However, we must still be wary of the messages presented to younger children.

There are a lot of people online who seem to think children are capable of making huge life decisions when they have barely started school. Let children be children, for fucks sake; they'll have plenty of time to make bad decisions later in life, as we all do. Above all else, we must eliminate one message, particularly when it's directed at children or other vulnerable individuals.

15

There's Something Wrong With YOU

This is essentially what someone is saying when using "the phrase" to another person. Lots of words spring to mind to use here, such as condescending, demeaning, and patronising, but I think I'll go with thoughtless and cruel. This is especially true if said to a child or someone with a permanent condition. Imagine being on the autism spectrum and hearing the phrase being repeated over and over. Receiving such a message from another person is bad enough, but this feeling must be intensified by its prevalence in all forms of media. Some of this messaging is obvious, but more often, it is done discreetly.

I rarely watch the news, never buy newspapers, and spend as little time online as I need to, yet I still tend to know what's going on in the world for the most part. In the pre-Internet era, evading politics, disasters, and advertising wasn't difficult if you wanted to. You could turn off the TV, not buy papers or magazines, and avoid anyone likely to be talking about them. You would now need to visit a remote location or wander about with your eyes closed and wearing ear defenders constantly. Although I'm sure it won't be long before you can hike to the most Northern part of our planet, only to find a sign saying, "The North Pole, Sponsored by… [probably some brown fizzy drink]".

The reality is that we are bombarded with advertising everywhere we look, and when it comes to online marketing, it is highly targeted to be specific to the individual. Even if you choose to opt out of "targeted ads" on your browser, profiles, and operating system, somehow, they mysteriously send you an ad connected with something you have recently discussed. This is not me being paranoid; I'm sure it's happened to you too. Please say it does, and I'm not being paranoid after all!

Here's a personal example: earlier this year, I shared the following on my Facebook timeline:

> You know how it's not a good idea to go online to check to see if you have certain conditions? Well, due to a couple of people over the last year asking whether I had ever been tested for ADHD, I went online today to do a test. The results came back positive. At the end of the test, there was a long description of causes, symptoms & treatments. I got bored reading it after a minute or so, & went to do something else. The test may be on to something!

Ever since sharing this, I see something connected to ADHD every time I go on the platform. Without fail, it will be one of the first things I see. This ranges from what may be causing it to what can sort it out, and as I said in the preface to this book, most of it is bollocks. There are also short videos or "reels" with people suggesting "this is what it is like to have ADHD" in particular situations. I've only watched a couple for research purposes, and surprise, surprise, the individuals in the videos were merely pretending to have, perhaps even mocking, the condition solely to attract more likes to their page.

Weirdly, though, I am still waiting to see a targeted ad after posting this:

> Experiment: My legs look great in a tutu. How long before I see an ad for such attire?!

Once upon a time, most advertising went along the lines of "Your life will be great as soon as you buy our product". This still exists, but there is definitely a rise in the "There's something wrong with you; you need our product" type of advertising. It's concerning enough that these types of ads are targeting vulnerable individuals, but what's even worse is that they are now aimed at children with messages suggesting that "if your child behaves in a certain way—essentially, like a child—then you need to purchase our product or service". This will reinforce the message to the child that "there's something wrong with you". This is why I believe it is essential to carefully consider the information we are exposed to, especially regarding children. At the same time, it's important not to do this in an overly protective manner, as society currently does by attempting to hide or ban things. When something becomes banned, curiosity kicks in, making us want to either find out why or try the thing if it is a substance. Smoking or vaping is an example of what parents try to ban children from doing, often unsuccessfully. It's one of the reasons I continued to smoke after being caught when I was a teenager.

Here are a couple of more banning failure examples:

- Prohibition of alcohol in the U.S. from 1920 to 1933. Well, that worked out fine, didn't it? Apparently, this is still practised in some towns and counties, but "alcohol-free" is not something that would spring to mind when I think of America.
- The "video nasties" of the late seventies and early eighties. Although tame by today's standards, seventy-two films were banned. This got people talking about and wanting to see them. This list included such titles as The Driller Killer (1979), Cannibal Holocaust (1980), and The Evil Dead (1981), all of which I managed to see a pirate copy of as a teenager.[33] [34] [35] It was only curiosity and wanting to know why they were banned that drove me to watch them. They would not have been on my radar otherwise.

It isn't feasible to protect a child from negative experiences, nor is it conducive to developing essential life skills. From what I've read in numerous sources, our analytical function does not begin to emerge until the age of six, which means that before this, information is assumed to be fact. Children have much more vivid imaginations than most adults, take things literally, and are just starting to develop their view of objective reality. In other words, they live in a fantasy world where they can be anything, and what that is can change daily. It is a mysterious and often contradictory world with lots of puzzles to solve. Every day in this world provides new experiences, some enjoyable and others upsetting. This is a time for playing and learning, not for making important decisions about who and what you are or will be.

When they grow up, and it's time for them to act responsibly and make their own decisions, we don't want them to be dependent on medication, have an unrealistic view of the world, or feel like there's something wrong with them. If most adults do not receive the help they need, it is vitally important that we do not create even more individuals who are incapable of solving their problems without medication or professional assistance. As we've seen, the odds are not stacked in your favour to get professional help to resolve an issue later in life, should one even try to.

16

You can Lead a Horse to Water...

Let's start this chapter by reversing one of the statistics I shared earlier from the World Health Organisation (page 56): three out of four people who would benefit from treatment do not receive it. Another way of looking at their number is that 72.4% of people suffer alone. It shouldn't be this way, and does not need to be either.

However, some people may recognise they have a problem and can be offered support, yet they are so entrenched in their ways that they refuse to make the changes that would benefit them. Not everyone will take their medicine. It is worth pointing out here that most medications are not a cure but rather a means of reducing the worst symptoms; the root cause of the problem still exists. When it comes to mental health, talking therapies can help facilitate the changes a person needs to make, but only the individual can make them. Sadly, even with the best intentions, you can't help everyone, only those who will allow you. Of course, many people do not even acknowledge that they have a problem. There is little point in offering advice until they can see it themselves. If you can see that a person has a problem, but they don't, sometimes you have to bite your lip or risk coming across as a Sheldon Cooper, or more accurately, if I'm to use fictional characters from *The Big Bang Theory*, a Beverly Hofstadter.[36] If I'm being brutally honest, I have done this more often than I'd like to admit.

Even when someone acknowledges they have a problem, they may still not want to discuss it, and if you persist, they are likely to snap at you. Here's one recent example: in a social setting, I regularly speak with an ex-Royal Marine who suffers from depression and PTSD. He has some other medical conditions and is in his seventies. A few years ago, I gave him a copy of my book for Veterans with PTSD. At the time, he seemed lifted and praised my book to other people. Due to the COVID-19 lockdowns, I didn't see him for a couple of years.

Recently, when I've seen him, he has either been so down that he didn't want to speak to anyone, preferring to be left alone, or in a highly agitated state, ranting about some issue related to the current state of politics. He had valid reasons to be outraged by many things, but why continue reading it if there's nothing you can do about it? I casually pointed out that if the news upset him so much, why not put the phone away? Circular reasoning came in as he said he enjoyed knowing what was happening. Here, I made my *Big Bang Theory* mistake of saying, "But do you?" His rage was then entirely projected onto me briefly as he impolitely suggested I stop doing my "psycho-shit". This was not my first rodeo, so diffusing the situation and moving onto a different topic without reacting emotionally myself was easy. If you don't know how to handle these situations, they can escalate quickly to a total relationship breakdown. That's not to say that I can't have my buttons pushed at times when I'm not in therapist mode. Oh yes, I can get triggered too!

Ultimately, only the individual can make changes for the better if they want to. Having covered some of the negative aspects of poor mental health, I'd like to share some potential options to feel good again. I nearly used the word OK there, but resisted. Although I just did, didn't I? Doh!

17

Complementary Therapists

Firstly, notice the word "complementary", meaning it works well in conjunction with something else. In other words, your first port of call should be your doctor; if you can get an appointment, that is! The health service here in the UK is underfunded, understaffed, and under pressure, even more so when it comes to mental health. If you can't get to see someone in the traditional sphere for six months or more, you might want to see someone complementary while waiting, but the choice is yours. I looked into the waiting list to get a diagnosis for ADHD for myself at the time of writing this book, and found it could be anywhere up to five years. Well, I made it to fifty-three, being the way I am, so I will not worry too much about it now. There are way too many people on waiting lists who deserve to be seen before me.

Numerous disciplines can help with mental health conditions, some more recognised than others, but what is most important is finding the right one for you. But please remember that all that these practitioners do is help you to help yourself. For example, I am classed as a “Hypnotist”, but a better description would be a “De-hypnotist” because what I used to do was help a client remove the bad mental programming that the influences on their life had hypnotised them with. I would love to credit the person I first heard use this term, but I can’t remember who it was. In more simple terms, I helped people to discover and remove the bullshit which had held them back.

Anyway, my point is that there are many options for you to explore, and many practitioners do a free initial consultation, which gives you a chance to see if it’s really for you. Trust your gut feeling rather than what others say about the discipline, and certainly not the therapist's claims. Be extremely careful when reading online reviews, too. Comments created by bots and fake accounts in comment sections of social media promotions usually follow a pattern that can easily be spotted if you read enough of them. There are also businesses that make their money by offering review services. I get plenty of emails every week, offering to drive my position higher up in Google rankings, increase my social media presence, and create “real” customer reviews. There was a time when I would have probably taken them up on their offer, except I always figured that an email from an unexpected source would be a scam, so I didn’t. Nowadays, I am not that interested in where I rank on Google or any other platform. If I am to have online reviews saying how fucking awesome, I am, I want them to be genuine. If you were to look for my online reviews at the time I am typing this, you would not find many, if any. In early 2024, I had a purge of most of my online presence, including deleting my Facebook business page, which had around 3000 followers. I hadn't shared that much and wanted a fresh start. Besides, most of my work with clients has been in the real world, so I preferred to have referrals to reviews. A good review is great, but clients put cash in your pocket.

The key takeaway here is not to place your faith, and more importantly, your mental health, in someone else's hands simply because they have thousands of reviews. The best therapists are not necessarily the most well-known, nor does price guarantee results. That's not to say that some famous expensive ones aren't good, and if you can afford to see one, you might as well give it a shot. Although it always tickles me when I see someone's marketing claiming to be "The World's Best…" "The UK's No.1…" or other made-up nonsense.

Why do I say nonsense?

- Well, how was this accolade given?
- Who were the judges?
- When and where was the competition held?
- And where the fuck was my invite!

I joke; I was a good therapist, but I'm under no delusion that I was the best. There are many other good therapists out there that you've never heard of, either. I'm sure many of them would be grateful for the business. There will also be many relatively new people who could do with the experience. To give you an idea of how many therapists there are, contemplate this: I placed an advert in the Hypnotherapy section of the Yellow Pages when I started working at a Health Centre in 1999. If you are asking yourself, “What the fuck is the yellow pages?” don’t worry about it. It is unimportant if you are too young to remember paper directories. If it bothers you, Google it.

So, way back in the last millennium, there were three paid ads in the Hypnotherapist section, including mine, and about eight others who merely had the free ad with name, address and telephone number. Ten years later, when I left the centre, there were three full pages with a mixture of paid and free ads. That was fifteen years ago, and since then, cheap online courses have been advertised everywhere. I am honestly surprised that there is anyone who isn’t trained in some discipline by now.

Even going to see a poorly trained novice could benefit you by the mere fact that you can get some shit off your chest. During my depression, I saw a CBT therapist and an NHS counsellor, and the main thing I got out of it was the chance to let off some of the pressure from all the shit going on in my head. A bit of a rant here and there did wonders, even though when it came to any specific advice they’d give, I usually thought, “Yeah, I know”. If you’re British and over thirty, please tell me that when you read that last quote, you heard it in your mind in Matt Lucas’ voice!

What I am about to share will, technically speaking, be my least ethical advice in this book; however, my sincere hope is for you to experience a genuine improvement in your well-being. When I say this idea might be unethical, I mean it may be considered to lack integrity by some, but that’s it; it won’t cause any actual harm to anyone. So here it is; with so many therapists offering “free initial consultations”, like I used to do, you could visit as many therapists as you like and not pay a single penny. Of course, there would be no continuity as such. Although rare, I did occasionally help someone get over a debilitating concern in one of these free 30-minute sessions. Having more than one of these freebies may be all you need. If money is tight and therapy is a luxury you can't afford, it's something to consider. On the other hand, if you can afford it, pay. Ripping people off may benefit your bank balance, but it is another indicator of poor mental health, by this book's definitions at least.

When you're suffering with your mental health, it is not easy to seek help, I know, I've been there, but honestly, it will be worth making the effort. Even if you don't want to go for any ongoing treatment, just speaking to someone once will give you a significant mental boost. If talking to someone face to face doesn't appeal, there are always online or telephone services to consider, such as the Samaritans. If getting help directly still doesn't do it for you, you could always consider getting some training.

18

Therapist Training

Here's a little thing you might not know about people who become therapists: generally speaking, they need therapy, too. It is said this is what draws them to the profession. I've met a few who are less enlightened than they tried to make out for sure. Another profession that attracts people with psychological problems to it is acting. I have trained as both, so read into that what you will!

As mentioned in the previous chapter, many cheap courses are available online. I can't comment on how good they are, but I know from a reliable source that someone offers good practitioner-level courses for about seven dollars. To put this in perspective, I paid £200 in 1997 (around $330 at the time) for an N.L.P. correspondence course.

You don't need to want to become a therapist to train as one. Just think about this: at the bare minimum, you will likely pay four times the cost of one of these seven-dollar courses for a single C.B.T. session. Instead of being given an exercise to try, you can learn all of them and try them out to see what works for you. You could also offer suggestions to friends and family who might find them useful.

A discipline I am trained in, which I found to be very effective, is called E.F.T., which stands for Emotional Freedom Techniques. It is relatively easy to learn compared to studying a talking therapy like C.B.T. or N.L.P. I was highly sceptical of the efficacy of a "tapping technique" when I first attended the in-person training, but was soon blown away by its ability to work on conditions so quickly. In 2011, I participated in a tandem skydive despite a fear of heights to demonstrate its effectiveness when writing my previous book. To put this in perspective, I've suffered an attack of vertigo when just wearing a VR headset! On the day of the jump, I used purely E.F.T. to enable me to go through with it with very little anxiety. I have to say, it was a fucking incredible experience.

There are so many disciplines you could train in that can help reduce the symptoms associated with mental health, and there are many businesses offering training. For the most part, it remains an unregulated industry, despite all the letters that can be promised to accompany your name upon completing your training. As I've mentioned many times before, do your research first. Look for a skill that appeals to you, then look into who offers training at a price you can afford. If you plan to do some training and turn it into a profession, please consider that trying to get clients and establish yourself brings a whole new stress load.

Here are just a few of the things you'll need to consider:

- Sales and marketing
- Dealing with cancellations and no-shows

- Being prepared for quiet periods with no clients
- Taking bookings
- Keeping financial records
- Keeping secure client notes
- Being compliant with data protection laws
- Getting professional liability insurance
- Finding somewhere to practice from

Many complementary therapists do not make their living solely from offering their services. Some come from two-income families where the therapist is basically pursuing a paid hobby. Others, like myself, have had to do other regular work to be sure to pay the bills every month, with the therapy money being for life's little extras. Sometimes, it irked me when I thought of the time and money I had spent on training and studying, only to have to do menial jobs to support myself. However, the experiences I gained from this and what I learned firsthand about human behaviour at all levels of society cannot be found in a book. I spent three years driving a taxi, a decade working in prisons, and in 2019, I even dressed as a female mouse to entertain children at a theme park for minimum wage! Although the latter job was done when I hoped to make a living as an actor and filmmaker. Don't let any of this put you off from doing some training and pursuing a career in therapy. Yes, many people don't succeed, but some certainly do; perhaps you will be one of them.

19
Self-Help

There are many branches of psychology, psychotherapy and talking-type disciplines on offer, with practitioners being of the belief that they have the answers to how the mind works. They will agree on certain principles and totally disagree on others. All of them get good results with clients, but also experience failures. With this being the case, the people involved in the process must be more accountable for results than the technique itself. By this, I mean the client and the professional they are working with. Even within the same field, two therapists may disagree on the likely cause of a condition.

Having read books on many of these theoretical frameworks, I am more convinced than ever that nearly all forms of healing and improvement can be classified as self-help, at least in terms of mental health. Practitioners merely help the individual themselves to facilitate the change using various methods. The blockages holding us back are removed or highlighted to enable the required healing or breakthrough.

Typically, self-help conjures the idea of tackling challenges independently. Working on your problems alone will take longer than working with a professional, but this is the only realistic option for some people. Thoroughly researching your condition from various sources, including videos and books, and attending in-person events requires considerable time. Notice I didn't say the internet as a source. This is because although you can find the information you need, you will also encounter a lot of nonsense that will make you worse. If you're going to use the internet, be very discerning with the info you come across. You should be open-minded and try things to see what works for you, but be wary of scammers.

Many things I've overcome in life have come from going down this often-lonely route. This is primarily why I decided to start writing short books that anyone can easily understand and only take a few hours to read at most. I want to help people who, like me, by necessity, have to slug it out alone for the most part. If this is you, I want to get you started on the journey with a few simple suggestions you might want to try. I say simple, but that doesn't mean they will be easy.

20

7 Simple Ways to Improve Your Mental Health

All seven suggestions to enhance your mental well-being are entirely optional, but just having a crack at one of them will benefit you, I assure you. Even with a severe condition, any improvement must be worthwhile, right? The more ideas you implement, the more significant the improvements will be, and they are just a starting point for you to begin a journey of mental transformation. Fuck, that last sentence sounded cringeworthy and gimmicky, didn't it? I'll still leave it in because, however sickly and overused the sentiment is, it just so happens to be true.

A minority of the readers of this book may embrace all seven ideas and experience an almost miraculous transformation in their lives, which would be fantastic if it does occur. However, most people will think about doing it but never bother: the "I'll start tomorrow" excuse. This is sad but undeniably true. Most people just can't be arsed to do the things which will improve their situation. The number of positive suggestions I have personally implemented is dwarfed by comparison to the many I am aware of, so don't feel bad if you do the same. The remaining few readers will pick one or two ideas that they like or that "resonate with them", to use the correct buzz term. They will work on them and start to see gradual progress. As their well-being improves, they will begin to look to gain more control over other aspects of their lives. Anything is truly possible when this level of responsibility is reached, so it is said. Of course, there will also be some people who think all these tips are a load of bollocks. Which of these four types will you be? If nothing else, based on what I've said about social media throughout this book, at least give the first suggestion a go.

1) Put The Bloody Phone Away!

I have a brother who is 20 years my junior, and I must say this to him nearly every time I see him. We could be out in the countryside walking my dog, watching a movie at the cinema, or round at our Mums for Sunday dinner. Even if he puts it away, you can guarantee it will be back out within less than a minute. Pointing out that one day he will look up from his phone and we'll no longer be there doesn't change his behaviour. Congratulations, bro, you made it into my book, although I imagine you will only see this if it somehow gets shared on your phone!

Having a device that has this much control over you is not healthy. If you are like this, it might be time for you to conduct a social media reset. You've probably come across this advice before, possibly contemplated it, and you know it makes sense. Social media is a big part of life nowadays, and some adults will not remember when it didn't exist. I imagine that just reading the section heading will have caused a slight dread for some people. If it was only a little bit of stress, then a reset, or as some describe it, a detox, is definitely for you. On the other hand, some are addicted to social media in a very similar way to how an alcoholic is addicted to booze. That is, the very thought of going without will cause a severe anxiety flare-up. I'm not going to suggest that anyone needs to quit social media, but if you believe you can't live without it, I highly recommend seeing a professional. It is not my intention to deal with complex problems like addiction in this book.

From everything I've said, it may seem like I'm against social media, but this is not the case; I have a neutral view of it. Just like an axe can be used to chop wood or be wielded by a homicidal maniac, I think social media is just another tool that can be used for both good intentions and ill. Like any tool, it should be used as required and then put away. You wouldn't walk around looking at a hammer all day after knocking a nail in, would you? Would you? If so, you might want to consider your life choices seriously. I jest, but is looking at a load of nonsense for hours a day a good use of your limited time on the planet? By the way, I've been just as guilty as the next person of spending far too long simply scrolling and scrolling. It still happens occasionally, but very rarely, I'm pleased to say. However, I am annoyed with myself when I do.

If you want to improve your mental health, spend some time working out what your personal social media reset should look like. Decide which bits you need and which bits you don't. Keeping in touch with contacts is useful, for example.

At the time of writing, AI is being used to create some very believable images and videos on all manner of topics, from ancient history to celebrity gossip and politics, which is an absolute load of bullshit. Knowing this, how do you tell fact from fiction? Not easily is the answer. Anybody can be cloned by AI now, including you. We have freely provided all the information necessary to do this for years. How many pictures of you are there online, and which years do they cover? I would guess there are, at least, hundreds of images of you from nearly every angle. If you've ever participated in a "then & now" picture challenge, there's a good chance your likeness spans a sufficient period for AI to determine how you appeared and will appear at any age. If you've ever been in a shared video where you are talking, there's your voiceprint, all ready to go.

Using social media to find out what is happening in the world regarding personally important topics falls into the category of "not useful" as far as I'm concerned. Hootsuite states, "On average, more than one billion fake Facebook accounts are removed each quarter".[37] Each of these fake accounts is trying to manipulate people in some way. You wouldn't want to put up with it in real life, so don't accept it from total strangers online. None of us likes to admit to being hoodwinked; it makes us feel stupid. This is why some will still stick to their convictions even when presented with undeniable evidence. Pick any political leader from any party, and plenty of false information will be spread about them online. If they are not the person you support, you are likelier to believe negative information about them than anything about the leader you support. It's both sad and amusing to enlighten someone to some truth only to hear, "Well, it's the kind of thing they might do!"

I sincerely recommend that you view everything, and I do mean EVERYTHING, that you view online with a critical and cynical eye. This is especially true regarding things that support your current beliefs on any subject. The algorithms are set up to show you more of what you appear to be interested in. These algorithms are also set up to show you more things that upset you than brighten your day, or so it seems to me. In other words, you're more likely to see a fake news article than a cat video.

This is how I endeavour to treat ALL information when I first come across it, whether it be online or elsewhere; feel free to try it on for size:

> As I wasn't there and don't have access to all the related data, I am unable to accept this as fact. Therefore, it is only logical to keep an open mind. What I am looking at is likely biased or untrue, so I'll file it as fictional entertainment. Without further reliable proof, I will not allow it to alter my emotional state negatively.

As part of the reset, I suggest taking at least one day off each week from these types of distractions and establishing a daily time limit for your online activities. You don't need to do it immediately; you can build up to it slowly if you need to. I've gone weeks without visiting social media, and do you know what I missed? Go on, have a guess. The answer will be after the following paragraph.

If your work involves being online, you may not be able to take long periods away from the internet, but if it does, avoid the temptation to have a "quick look, it won't hurt" moment. Speaking from experience, "quick" usually turns into a more extended session than a planned one. Even those times when you are technically skiving off and getting paid to look at nonsense, I'd recommend reading a book instead. Some jobs genuinely demand that we are contactable when on-call, but does yours, really? If it doesn't involve life and death decisions, I'd suggest the answer is no.

Fuck All! That is the answer to what I missed out on during a long break from social media. Did you guess correctly? FOMO, the Fear of Missing Out, is irrelevant if you consider it. On Facebook alone, there are over a billion new posts per day, so you'll miss out on something whether you like it or not. Just knowing about something for knowing's sake is extremely unlikely to benefit you in any tangible way, and quite possibly the opposite regarding your mental well-being. Does knowing that someone has become famous for talking about spitting on a penis have any real bearing on your life? Only you can answer that question. This was a highly talked-about thing in 2024. When I finally watched the video in January 2025, because curiosity got the better of me, I didn't find it particularly funny. I guess that's because you hear far cruder and entertaining conversations when you've lived in a confined space on a warship with fifty other sailors!

None of us knows how much time we will have in this life. Those under thirty tend not to give much thought to this idea. Between thirty and fifty, individuals become aware, yet they likely still believe that they will enjoy a long lifespan and that early death only occurs to others. After fifty, the slightest pain, and you think it's game over, man!

With age comes wisdom, so it is said. It's slightly annoying to work some vital shit out and then think, why didn't I do this years ago. The sooner somebody realises how much of their limited time is being wasted, the more likely they are to live a fulfilling life. So, contemplate this for a moment: the average person sleeps for four months of the year and spends a further three months at work, including travelling time. This leaves just five months for everything else we do. Eating, bathing, and time spent on the toilet must take away at least another month. Two hours a day spent on any particular task equates to one more month per year gone. Does pointless scrolling and swiping to merely pass the time still seem appealing to you?

When a person's sands of time are nearly run out, and they are lying on their deathbeds, they often reflect upon their lives and contemplate any regrets. When it's your turn, will your time spent on social media be something you consider to have been valuable? Or, do you think you would wish you had spent that time more productively? In the unlikely event that you should think it was a good use of time, will you have spent it mostly being supportive or unsupportive?

2) Does Pineapple Belong on Pizza?

You undoubtedly have an opinion on this question, but I don't; I don't like tomatoes, so I don't eat pizza. But to bring us back to social media once more, this question is a good example of the point I wish to make.

You will see more posts on this question from those who are against the idea than those who are for it, am I right? Pick any topic, and you will see the same pattern: more people ranting about what they are against. This can be trivial things like pizza toppings, hanging your bogroll correctly, or whether a particular TV show is shite. This idea extends to significant issues, including foreign aid, immigration policies, and political candidates in elections. I hesitate to categorise this as serious, but it also pertains to the debate over whether the Earth is round or flat. It is a topic that gets much coverage from many celebrity scientists, such as Neil deGrasse Tyson. Most of these videos attack the flat Earth model rather than promote the truth. The number of videos supporting the flat Earth stance pales in comparison. Is this truly a good use of Neil and Co.'s time and energy? Personally, I wouldn't want to waste my precious time on something that doesn't require an intelligent debate.

Whether you like or loathe him, it is safe to say that Donald Trump is the most controversial and divisive U.S. President in living memory, possibly ever. During his successful presidential campaigns and first term in office, my Facebook timeline was filled with comments that fit into the against category. A month into his second term, it has also proven to be the same case. You may think, "Well, all your friends must be anti-Trump!" This is not the case. As an adult, I choose to act like an adult and not a child, most of the time anyway. Therefore, I do not fall out with my friends based on their political beliefs. I have friends and family who lean to the left and others who lean to the right. Sometimes, when I read one of their posts, I think to myself, "What the fuck are you sharing, you fucking bellend?" This is especially true when such a post is easily verified as false. I'll sit in a state of disbelief for a few moments and then look for a good memory I have of the person. I never became friends with anyone because of politics; it was because of something we had in common. I may disagree with them over many things, but this can't be avoided, so I tend not to discuss the most contentious topics with anyone. If it's brought up, I will listen and try to determine why they feel this way. That is, unless I've had a few beers, in which case the soapbox may come out, accompanied by a good rant. However, no one changes their mind just because you call them a twat. I did want to use the "C" word there, but I promised at the start of this book that I wouldn't. If you completely shut out a person you know because of their beliefs, it will be impossible to help them see another perspective.

Here's the critical question for this tip: What emotions do you feel when spending your time and energy on something you are against? I'll wager they are the same emotions people feel when their mental health is poor, by my definition. Don't you think it's insane to voluntarily spend your day sharing an opinion that causes you to feel bad, knowing it will make zero difference to anyone but you? I must also be insane, for I still do it, albeit extremely rarely and nowhere near as frequently as before I heard a quote attributed to Mother Teresa. In a YouTube video of the late Dr Wayne Dyer, he mentioned that she was invited to attend an anti-war rally, which she declined, saying she would gladly participate in a pro-peace Rally. It may seem odd because it's essentially the same desired outcome. That is, until you realise what she was getting at. She did not want to give any energy to what she was not for, in this case, war. Now, think of something you are actually for and how you feel when doing something towards that end. I bet the emotions you think of are all positive, right? So here comes a rhetorical question: if you want to feel better, should you spend more time and energy on the things you are for or those you are against?

As I said at the start of these tips, they're simple but not necessarily easy. Changing a habit like this may take a while, but it is doable. Simply reflecting on what I've shared in this tip provides a strong starting point and puts you ahead of many individuals who may never even consider it.

The things we are against tend to endure for as long as people dedicate time and energy to them. When the balance shifts, they tend to disappear. If you've ever heard of the Law of Attraction, you should already understand the importance of this tip. If you haven't, I'll explain it quickly in overly simple terms, although I prefer the term Law of Deliberate Intent because the former term is often shared as if you can manifest a sports car just by thinking about it. I have had many strange coincidences, or more accurately synchronicities, occur based upon intention. However, I have yet to manifest an Aston Martin DBS by simply thinking about it, so I still drive an eighteen-year-old car! In essence, these laws suggest that our predominant thoughts and feelings tend to manifest in our lives. There's a lot more to it, lots of people talking about it, and quite a few that suggest they can help you manifest your heart's desires, for a price, of course. My research so far seems to indicate that by the time your consciousness reaches this point, many of these wanted items are no longer desired. But, for now, I wouldn't get overly concerned with any manifestation techniques until you're on top of your mental health.

According to this theory, though, the people who opposed Donald Trump's election and focused so much of their time, energy, and thoughts on him were just as responsible for this becoming a reality as those who were actually for him. If you are heavily into a political party, it's something to think about in the future.

If you are wondering about my political beliefs, I'll just say that I'm not interested in supporting either side in a two-party system like we currently have in the UK. This type of politics tends to be primarily confrontational and is more focused on "you're wrong" than looking for solutions to problems. Neither side can solve all the issues we face to everyone's satisfaction. I am not one of those who think all politicians are the same. There is a lot of corruption and pocket-lining going on, which became very evident during the 2020 pandemic. There are also people on both sides of the political spectrum who genuinely want to do right by their country. Maybe, if politicians were only paid the "living wage", we'd attract more of this type of person. That about sums up my political viewpoint, so let's move on.

Changing to being a person who focuses on what they stand for won't be easy because you'll be going against the norm. Friends and family will share what they are against, and the temptation to join the conversation will be intense. The impact of your sharing your opinion will probably be negligible, at best, on the discussed topic, but it will get you in some type of agitated state. Avoiding saying anything may not make much difference to how you feel because you'll still be thinking about it. However, if I were still a betting person, I would confidently wager that your mental health would improve if you regularly share what you are for, provided it is done in a non-antagonistic manner. I don't mean in the pompous "I'm a Vegan" kind of way, for example. While I'm not a vegan, I fully support anyone who adopts a vegan lifestyle; however, I'm not fond of the preachy attitude some exhibit.

As the saying goes, "Misery loves company"; if that's your predominant way of feeling, don't be surprised when you get more of it. The converse is also true, so try putting your thoughts and actions into what you are for, and fuck what anyone else thinks.

3) Humour IS Your Greatest Ally

Motivating yourself to do anything can be extremely difficult if you're feeling low. I get it; I've been there. I've had days where depression has kicked in for no apparent reason, and I have sat on the couch having an internal repetitive dialogue along the lines of:

Logical Therapist Voice: Come on, all you need to do is get up and start doing anything, and you'll begin to feel better.

Victim Voice: Fuck off! I know that, but I just can't right now.

Logical Therapist Voice: Come on, you know you want to, really.

Victim Voice: If I could, I would, but I can't, so I shan't.

Logical Therapist Voice: (reverse psychology) Stay there feeling sorry for yourself, then.

Victim Voice: Thanks, I will. P.S. Fuck you; I know what you're trying to do.

This back and forth could last minutes or sometimes hours, but at some point, I would have to move, even if it was just to let the dog out. If it were a long spell, I would explore the dark feelings and see where they'd take my thinking, almost like watching a movie from a detached perspective. However, the thing which could nearly always lift my mood was comedy. Some days, even turning on the TV felt impossible, and it took hours to manage it. The sooner I acted, the better it was for my mental state because we cannot feel opposing emotions simultaneously. No matter what type of humour you enjoy, when you are engrossed in it and have a good belly laugh, even if it's only for a short time, it's impossible to feel low in this state.

If you serve in the military, you tend to develop a vast sense of humour that can range from childish to very dark, likely by design, as it helps you to get through the shit times. No matter the situation, there would always be someone who could find a way to put a humorous spin on it. In the lower ranks, certainly in the Navy at least, a lot of the peacetime working day is spent taking the piss out of each other and winding someone up to see if you can get a rise. If they "bite", they are instantly called on it, and most of the time, realise they've been had and laugh with you. Occasionally, you might get punched first, but that would just add to the delight of getting them. I'm not recommending this approach to life, but I hope you can see the value and power of humour. This is one of many reasons we Veterans struggle to fit back into regular civilian society. Civilians don't get how we can seem to take lightly many of the matters they consider serious. We just see their stern reaction as pomposity!

Quick question: Have you been keeping track of how many times I've used this word now?

An internet connection is all you need to access some of the best moments in comedy. Most of this content is available for free on YouTube, and DVDs can be found for very little money in charity shops. At a time when you are feeling good, create a list of your favourite comedies, and then check where you can find them easily. Look for everything from short sketches to stand-up shows to full-length features. Collect online memes that make you giggle whenever you see them, and maybe even print a few out. Write down a few of your favourite one-liners that always make you laugh when you think of them, then find the clip of it being performed. For example, no matter how often I see it, the classic line from Eric Morecambe, "I'm playing all the right notes, but not necessarily in the right order", has me in stitches.[38] Even as I typed it, I pictured the scene and heard his voice saying it, and tears came to my eyes as I chuckled.

Stock up your comedy survival kit now; it could make a massive difference to your mental health. In fact, go and do it now whilst it's fresh in your mind and return when you've done it. Only if you want to, though; it's not an order!

4) The Truth IS "Out There"!

This was the tagline in the opening credits of the popular TV series *The X-Files*, which can convey at least a double meaning.[39] Firstly, in the sense that if you are determined to find the truth, it is there somewhere, and it's possible to discover it. Secondly, the truth can be far weirder than you imagined. Both of these interpretations can be applied to improving both your physical and mental health, but it is the latter interpretation I wish to discuss now.

There is nothing wrong with a bit of healthy scepticism, but approaching things with the dogmatic viewpoint of "This doesn't fit in with my beliefs" can prevent you from finding the truth. This idea resonates with a variety of scientists and many people of faith. We can see how religions have been used historically to control the masses to behave in particular ways. Most Wars, the crusades, and the persecution of non-conformists all fell under the banner of "Our truth is the ONLY truth", resulting in millions of deaths to make a few people extremely rich. However, except for anti-science advocates, most assume all scientists approach research subjects without personal biases. This is certainly not the case, and all the negative traits that can be associated with any hierarchical group apply to the world of science, too. Although aware of this for many years, to what extent this viewpoint holds back science was only recently confirmed when I read Rupert Sheldrake's *The Science Delusion*.[40] Before dismissing an idea as pseudoscientific, you would think they would at least read the research data. Much research has been carried out under strict control measures, which indicate support for many subjects considered to be a bit "woo-woo" by mainstream science. As a bit of a tangent within a tangent, I'd like to share that I once wrote in a blog post that "woo-woo" is simply an acronym for "Weird Occurrences Others Will Often Ostracise." Just putting it in print to prove I came up with it, should it ever catch on!

Maintaining an open mind tends to benefit the individual and all of humanity. It was the closed minds that, throughout history, held back progress and even persecuted freethinkers. Our understanding of the universe and many modern luxuries we take for granted are thanks to those who employed an open mind and ignored the naysayers. So, I always like to keep an open mind when it comes to improving mental and physical health. If the scientific community says that, under control conditions, a particular methodology is no more effective than a placebo, I would still give it a try. If you are unfamiliar with the placebo effect, simply put, it is when someone is given a sugar pill but believes it is an actual medication, and yet they still get better. Placebo surgery has even been carried out successfully, as mentioned in Bruce Lipton's fascinating book, *The Biology of Belief*.[41]

Does it matter if it's a specific crystal, herb, or your belief in its effectiveness that has brought about an improvement? I think the resulting improvements are the priority, don't you? We now have access to healing methods from across the globe, many dating back thousands of years. Stories of miraculous healings defy the scientific model and are often put down to mass hypnosis, but the healings still happen all the same. It's your health, so any final decision on what method to use is up to you. It's also essential to avoid the either-or approach in any case. Some individuals dismiss conventional Western treatments for a condition, believing that an alternative alone will suffice, often to their tragic detriment. A person's level of consciousness, which I alluded to in a previous chapter, could be a significant influencing factor in the effectiveness of a technique for both patients and practitioners.

5) Self-Development with a Capital "S"

This is a topic deserving of its own book, one that I plan to write at some point, so I will strive to keep this to just a few pages. If I haven't ruffled any feathers so far, this idea is bound to.

The phrase "Self with a capital S" frequently arises in personal and spiritual development discussions. It denotes your spirit, soul, or vital essence—the true core of who you are, distinguishing this from the everyday "self with a little s"- a temporary existence primarily focused on bodily concerns and gratifications. You will undoubtedly have a strong opinion about this already, and I am not here to convert anyone to any particular way of thinking. We are merely having a conversation to explore a topic which is and should be highly personal. If participating in such a discussion is not for you, that's all cool; just move on to the next tip on page 112 and imagine there are only six suggestions in this section. The last thing I want you to do is to decide this book is a load of shite because of a few pages that might contradict a firmly held belief. If you are happy to employ an open mind and suspend judgment and personal biases, I will share some observations.

People with regular religious or spiritual practices tend to be less prone to stress than the average person. These practices must be by personal choice, not because they are expected. I am not going to back this up with any more statistics. Many easy-to-find scientific studies on health and well-being have focused on meditators and similar groups, if you don't want to take my word for it. Throughout human history, an individual's religious or spiritual beliefs would have been dictated by place of birth and family tradition. Those in power could use this fact to benefit the entire group, tribe or geographical district. They could also impose strict rules and designate enemies, and the unscrupulous could make huge profits. This is still mostly the case today. The primary difference we have now is that anyone with an internet connection can learn about other paths and faiths. You no longer need to be wealthy, highly educated or have access to a physical library to educate yourself. If you take the time to do this, as I have done, the similarities of core teachings will jump out and slap you in the face. In addition to studying texts, I have attended many ceremonies and rituals based on various beliefs. I have practised meditation alongside Hindus and Buddhists, participated in several Native American Sweat Lodges, and attended ceremonies for Druid, Wiccan, and Thelemic traditions. At each of these events, I did not feel like an outsider; in fact, I felt safer and more welcome than at any other time in my everyday life.

We no longer need to fall for the "they've got it wrong and are evil" propaganda of the past. Anyone who preaches hate, no matter their denomination, is acting contrary to the teachings of the originator of them. I can't imagine Jesus would have approved of the Crusades, the Spanish Inquisition, or the slaughter of millions of indigenous people when Europeans arrived in the Americas. Words from different languages across the globe are used to express the same spiritual concepts of harmony and cooperation that the founders of these belief systems imparted. This cannot be a coincidence.

The atheist reading this section will probably be thinking, "Here we go, this book was not bad until this fucking bit, what a balloon!" That is a fair comment; you will no doubt consider yourself a student of science. I do, too, and I thought of myself as an atheist for a couple of years, but that was a long time ago, in a …! Woah, steady there, Stuart. Is this a Starwarsian slip, a random tangent, or are you going somewhere with this? I am going somewhere with it. This surprises me as I write this, as much as it might surprise you, the reader. In the *Star Wars* universe, numerous droids act as though they are humans, C3PO, for example. Although highly intelligent, it has no free will and relies on complex software design for its behaviour. It is a mechanical being incapable of doing anything which contradicts its programming. As an atheist who believes solely in the scientific materialism model, one has to, therefore, consider oneself to be nothing more than a droid. Is this how you perceive yourself? Do you honestly believe that the music which you absolutely fucking love is merely down to the reaction of chemicals in the body and the firing of particular neurons? If you do, good on you, but this doesn't sit right with me. The *Star Wars* analogy I just shared was not planned and just seemed to write itself; I find it hard to put that down to simple biology.

Many people in Western countries profess to belong to a particular religion, yet do not practice its teachings. The history of Christianity and its many different denominations has resulted in a heavy trail of bloodshed. This is not what Jesus taught, although it could be argued that he wasn't a Christian. The interpretations of the teachings of these prophets and Sages are often written long after their death. They can be easily misinterpreted either by accident or for political purposes. England is considered a Christian country, but this is done chiefly nowadays via lip service and more concerning Nationalism than faith. In America, there is often a pick the bits which back what you want to say approach to Christianity, with most of that coming from the Old Testament and not the teachings of Christ. In recent years, this has been utilised to alter or establish several controversial laws, despite the Constitution's First Amendment declaring that there shall be no official religion and that all citizens are free to follow any faith. Unsurprisingly, droves of people spot the hypocrisy in all this. When individuals realise this, they tend to do one of two things. They may become atheists and turn their backs on all forms of spirituality. Alternatively, they may develop an interest in beliefs from other parts of the world, which appear more harmonious and congruent with their teachings. In most countries, it still remains unusual for a person to distance themselves from familial beliefs and forge their own path. In the UK, the number of individuals identifying with the state religion has declined between censuses, with more than 100,000 people reporting adherence to a pre-Christian tradition in the 2021 census. Only 46.2% of the population declared themselves Christian, with 37.2% saying they had no religion.[42] As a percentage of the population, there are more Christians in America, which has no state religion, than in the UK, which is classed as a Christian country![43]

If you are fortunate enough to live in a place with religious freedoms, actively seeking to deepen your spirituality will likely positively impact your mental health. This could be through the religion of your family, one that calls to you, or a solitary investigation with no formal structure. If this search leads to a belief that supports life without condemning others, you will probably be on the right path.

6) Do Something for Someone Else

At the time of writing this page, I have begun creating a series of videos titled "Pay It Forward," abbreviated as "PIF," in which I share some personal development tips. The idea is sound, but whether I actually share them depends on how they turn out. It's weird how I have no problem being in front of a camera as an actor, but I am not so keen when I have to be me.

Any videos I create will be on my Website, YouTube channel and Facebook page only, should you be interested in finding them. If you see them anywhere else, it wasn't me that put them there, not that it matters. The concept behind this idea is that if a viewer finds the advice beneficial, they will reciprocate by doing something helpful for someone else; that is, they will pay it forward. They are welcome to share the video if they wish, but I would prefer that they also engage in other activities or at least do this as well. This might sound counterintuitive, even a little crazy, so let me explain my reasoning. Almost everything shared on social media is trying to get you to like it to boost the poster's ego or generate some money for them; probably both. I'm usually no exception regarding my business pages, but I'm fine if just one person appreciates any of the videos in this series. I don't care if they don't follow my page or ever buy a thing from me. Obviously, it would be even nicer if more people liked them, but that is not my intention. We all get upset when we share something we think is amazing, and then there is little interaction with it, especially when we see some of the absolute shite that goes viral. In this specific case, I will not be concerned in the slightest. Knowing that one person finds any of my videos in this series helpful will provide a rewarding feeling that only comes from helping others without expecting anything in return. This may sound like some hippy shit, but think about it for a moment. When you give a gift to someone you deeply care for, how do you feel as they begin to open it? Can you put that feeling into adequate words to describe it? I can't because "good" doesn't really do the feeling justice. I know I am not alone in feeling this way. In a recent UK YouGov poll titled *Agree or Disagree: I enjoy giving more than receiving presents*, 75% of 597 respondents said "agree".[44]

Although it may not be as intense, we can feel similar when we let someone out before us when driving, and they acknowledge us. If you've never done that because you're always in a rush to get to your destination, give it a try to see if I'm lying or not. It might be good for your blood pressure, too. We can also get this sensation when we help a stranger shorter than us to get an item from the top shelf in a supermarket. You get the idea, right?

Assisting another person or animal in distress when no one else will know you've done it evokes this weird, feel-good emotion in us. This simple deed can often brighten the rest of your day, and things that may have otherwise irritated you go unnoticed. This feeling is not to be confused with the one experienced by someone who does such things while being purposely filmed to share the deed online. This feeling may be nice, but it is short-lived because it is merely ego gratification. The pleasure the fragile ego receives soon passes, and it needs to find another emotional fix as quickly as possible. You've seen the videos; you know what I'm talking about. Would you tend to categorise these people as mentally healthy or slightly neurotic? If such a person's happiness is dependent on being popular and liked online, it means it can easily and quickly be turned into depression when they are no longer followed or relevant. Ultimately, happiness is an internal state that requires no external stimuli; we just tend to think it does.

Helping others distracts us from our own problems and provides a positive experience that enhances our mental health. People high up on the aforementioned consciousness scale help others as part of their life purpose. They are few and far between, so you do not have to try to emulate that level of dedication. Nevertheless, the more positive actions you take, the better your mental health will become.

7) Remember This Image

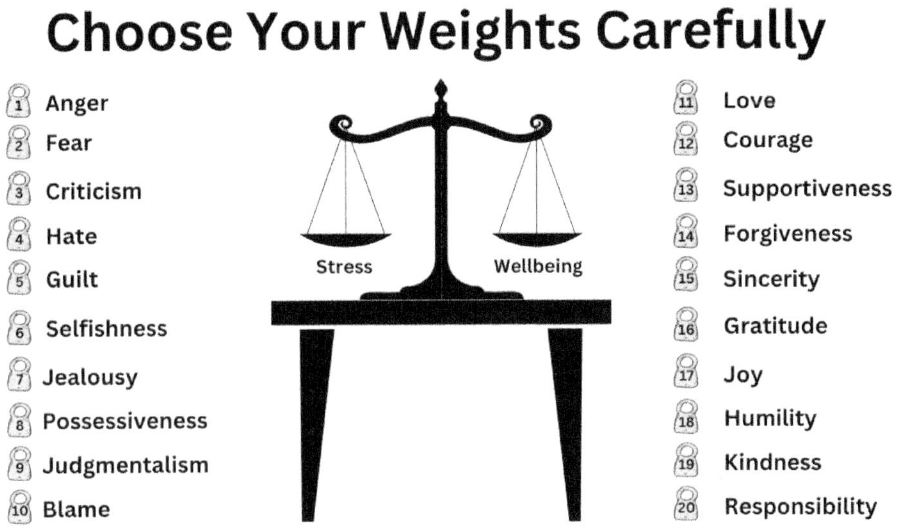

We are coming towards the end of our time together, and the end of this book is nigh. Unless you choose to reread it, much of what I've shared will be forgotten by you. This is why I left this tip until last; it will be the freshest in your memory. You may recall the parts of this book that evoked strong emotions, the parts that made you laugh, and the parts that pissed you off. I hope I managed to elicit these emotions at the right and intended moments. However, if you remember nothing else from reading this book, I want you to burn this image into your memory. You don't need to remember the names attached to each weight; they are simply examples of common behaviours. We all know that we should employ the weights from the right side of the image, but life sometimes makes us grab from the left. It's also the case that we are more likely to use the right-hand list with people we identify with. Using this list at all times, especially with people we dislike, is the real test of consciousness. As previously stated, not many achieve this level.

Your perception of the world, or personal reality, is partly formed in your brain from sensory experiences. Some of these experiences are real, others are imagined, but both have the same effect on your body.

Google Gemini provided the following quote, which is the only part of this book created using AI. For complete transparency, I also used Grammarly during the editing process to sort out some of my cock-ups. During this process, we had many differences of opinion when Grammarly wished to alter something, and I was adamant that I didn't!

> The autonomic nervous system (ANS) is a part of the peripheral nervous system that controls involuntary bodily functions. It has two main divisions:
>
> Sympathetic nervous system: Prepares the body for action, often known as the "fight-or-flight" response. It increases heart, blood, and breathing rates while decreasing digestion and other non-essential functions.
>
> Parasympathetic nervous system: Promotes rest and digestion, often known as the "rest-and-digest" response. It slows down heart rate, lowers blood pressure, and increases digestion.

These two systems work together to maintain homeostasis, the body's internal balance.[45]

That's nice, you may be thinking, but what the fuck does this have to do with your picture and my mental health? Good question. When people talk about the fight or flight response, they primarily focus on the "flight" side of it. There are many thousands of online articles and blog posts, most of which are carbon copies of each other, that will talk about how this anxious state is affecting your body physically. The "fight" part is rarely discussed in the same way. Anger management is mainly talked about in the context of extreme examples. However, sitting at a PC or staring at a phone and seething is equally affecting your physiology, too.

If you remember my analogy from an earlier chapter, you could say that the Murderous Beast completely controls your bodily functions when you are angry or anxious. It doesn't need to eat, doesn't need to shag, and doesn't have time to go for a shit right now. It is in a constant state of lookout for potential dangers. This is good when there is a real danger to your life. However, if there is no danger, it's better to let the Civilised Human take control of your body because it cares about all your systems running optimally. People with good mental health switch between the two states as is appropriate to a situation.

If we are thoroughly engrossed and suspend disbelief when we watch a scary movie, we will feel the same emotions as if the psycho killer is right there chasing after us. After the jump scare has occurred or the protagonist escapes their clutches, we get the release, and our Civilised

Human has a little laugh at our expense for waking the Beast unnecessarily.

Now, think about all the little movies you play in your mind all day, every day, and quite often, day after day. These are made up of memories of past hurts and future concerns. We all know we can't change the past, but that doesn't stop us from repeatedly playing these depressing old movies, does it?

We also do not know what the future holds for us; we may not even have that much of one for all we know, yet we can play movies in our minds about the worst possible scenarios that could happen in a situation. For example, if we were going on a first date, we might imagine everything that could go wrong. Since we won't know what will happen until we experience the date, wouldn't it be better to imagine the outcomes we want?

Let's tie this up now and show how it relates to the picture I want you to remember. Since the autonomic nervous system cannot differentiate between reality and vivid imagination, every movie we play in our minds influences our health. Whenever we feel a strong emotion, we add weight to one side or the other. There are no prizes for guessing which of the two pans you want to add the most weight to. We all have moments where we pick up weights from the negative list, but if the counterbalance is sufficiently stocked up, it will not have a long-term effect on our mental health. However, if we only add weight to the "stress" pan and then place a single weight on the "well-being" pan, it will seem as though nothing has changed. Nonetheless, it has made a difference by slightly reducing the weight required to start tipping the balance back in your favour. This is a solid beginning; simply continue increasing the weight on this side while ensuring you don't add any more to the other. The progress that can be made this way will vary from person to person and is a lifelong journey with no final destination other than the obvious one. However, there are as many resting spots as you need along the way.

Do not let this idea dishearten you because when I say it is an ongoing journey, I do not mean life will always seem a bit shitty. It is merely that even the people who inspire us will still pick up the wrong weights occasionally. The difference is that they have made sufficient progress, so their stress pan never carries excessive weight. I want this level of progress for you, and I hope you want it, too.

21

A World with Perfect Mental Health?

The pessimist will say this is impossible and probably agree with what Agent Smith from *The Matrix* had to say:

> As a species, human beings define their reality through suffering and misery. The perfect world was a dream that your primitive cerebrum kept trying to wake up from.[46]

Yeah, I have to concede that a mentally healthy world population isn't likely to happen in our lifetimes, but what would it look like if it did? As an optimist, I believe we are slowly evolving in the right direction, though it may take a million years or more for the entire human population to achieve perfect mental health. However, with each individual who enhances their mental health, there is a little less fear and hatred in the world. This is another small step in the right direction. Despite all the negative things I have said about social media and the internet, it cannot be denied that the number of people across the globe who desire this kind of future is growing. Like-minded individuals and groups are now able to connect easily. As this trend grows, some of the following things could become a reality within a couple of generations, while others will no doubt take a lot longer.

If all world leaders had good mental health, they would be able to resolve differences without invading other countries, and War would be a thing of the past, looked upon as an embarrassing and barbaric part of human evolution. These kinds of leaders would never consider a nuclear first-strike scenario. Anyone suggesting they would launch a first strike would never be allowed to hold that power, as it would lead to global annihilation. The money previously spent on destruction could be put into science projects that support life and expand our understanding of our planet, galaxy and universe. Sufficient resources would be available to guarantee quality education for all. Anybody choosing a political vocation would be motivated by a desire to improve conditions rather than power and wealth.

Without greed, starvation and disease could be swiftly addressed, and sufficient aid supplied when natural disasters strike. There would be enough to go around, and no one would go without what they need or want. With poverty eradicated, there would be no necessity to steal through any of the methods we currently encounter. On a planet with good mental health, murder, rape, and all other violent crimes would all but disappear, and potential perpetrators would be in the extreme minority. They could be recognised early and given appropriate treatment, support and education.

Problems concerning the environment and overpopulation could be discussed logically and scientifically, and reasonable and ethical solutions could be found. The imaginary borders created by man to divide the planet would no longer be necessary. Instead of fearing other cultures, we could learn from one another. We would accept that we are all uniquely different, with different tastes and desires. The individual could pursue their passions and dreams free from anxiety. It's fanciful stuff, I know, but that doesn't make it untrue.

I've mentioned the late comedian Bill Hicks a couple of times in this book, so I thought it fitting to end this chapter with an actual quote from one of his performances:

> Just a simple choice, right now, between fear and love. The eyes of fear want you to put bigger locks on your doors, buy guns, close yourself off. The eyes of love instead see all of us as one. Here's what we can do to change the world right now to a better ride. Take all that money we spend on weapons and defences each year and instead spend it feeding and clothing and educating the poor of the world, which it would pay for many times over, not one human being excluded, and we could explore space together, both inner and outer, forever, in peace.[47]

Wise words that he first uttered over thirty years ago. Globally, his message may appear to have had no impact, but many individuals will have looked at the world a little differently after hearing or reading it. I was one of these people. Will you be too?

22
Conclusion

I don't expect you to agree with everything I've said in this book, but I hope you agree that it is "Not OK to Be Not OK". As I pointed out a couple of times, being born with certain conditions does not make an individual any less of a person. In many cases, any ability which may be deficient in an individual is often compensated for by being exemplary in another. If this applies to you, never let anyone say you are "Not OK". I firmly believe that we all have greatness of some kind within us. This talent may be well hidden, and we may never uncover what it is; sometimes for lack of even looking for it. Being successful doesn't have to involve doing something that will bring you fame and fortune. The joy of simply doing it may be all you need to live a fulfilling life. Let's face it, lots of wealthy and/or famous people don't seem to be content with their lot in life. The thing which a person excels at doesn't have to be particularly grand or require a high IQ to make it meaningful. Academics possess specific skills, yet they will also be deficient in other areas where the uneducated might excel. If it is something which improves the lives of others, you enjoy doing it, and do it to the best of your ability, I would suggest you have found success.

Experiencing poor mental health is a normal and common part of life, but it is never OK; it is something that needs to be remedied as soon as possible. There are many ways to do this, and I have provided some examples. I will now summarise the best way to improve your mental health in one last bullet list:

- The antidote to your fears is to have the courage to step just outside your comfort zone into an unknown future.
- Your sadness will dissipate when you let go of the past and contemplate what a brighter future could look like.
- You will feel less agitated when you let go of any resentment towards others and yourself.
- Recognising that the only thing you truly have complete control over is your ability to change can help alleviate anger and irritation.
- Everybody has some goodness in them, even if it's only a little. This morality can grow, but only when it is acknowledged, so look for the good in other people and yourself.
- Remember: There is nothing wrong with you. You ARE Ok. We are all works in progress.
- You do not need to become a saint. We can all be a bit of a twat, so just work on being less of one today than you were yesterday!

There are many ways in which the world screws with your head, and I have only highlighted a few of them. Now that I have brought some of them to your attention, or more accurately, reminded you of them, you can look for others. You can reduce how often you are manipulated as you consciously spot them. It will still happen; it continues to happen to me, but the more control you regain for yourself, the better your overall mental health will be.

I'll end by reminding you of an important point. Life is full of ups and downs for everybody; there are good and bad times, but humour can help to get you through many of these things. While seriousness is sometimes necessary, it is often avoidable. The rest of the time, have fun and don't be afraid to act daft. We usually hold back because we worry about what others think of us. Well, as long as what you're thinking of doing isn't going to cause any harm, fuck what other people think. Let others exhibit their pomposity while you enjoy some silly moments!![48]

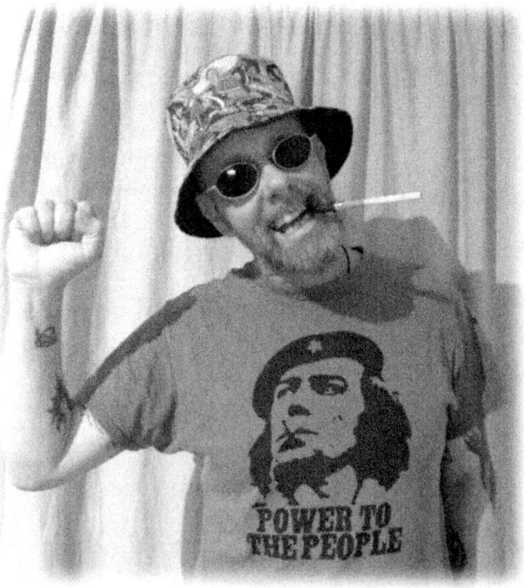

References

[1] Voltaire. 1930. Candide. Modern Library. New York.

[2] Bean, Sean. "Sharpe's Sword." Sharpe, season 1, episode 8, directed by Tom Clegg, aired December 18, 2024, on ITV.

[3] Carnegie, Dale, 1888-1955. 2009. How to Win Friends and Influence People. New York, Simon & Schuster.

[4] IHME, Global Burden of Disease (2024) – with minor processing by Our World in Data. "IHME GBD" [dataset]. IHME, Global Burden of Disease, "Global Burden of Disease - Deaths and DALYs" [original data].

[5] Gun violence archive (2025) Gun Violence Archive. Available at: https://www.gunviolencearchive.org/past-tolls (Accessed: 13 January 2025).

[6] The latest government data on school shootings (2024) https://usafacts.org/. Available at: https://usafacts.org/articles/the-latest-government-data-on-school-shootings/ (Accessed: 14 November 2024).

[7] Office for National Statistics (ONS), released 9 February 2023, ONS website, article, Homicide in England and Wales: year ending March 2022

[8] Stallone, S. (Director). (1982). First Blood [Film]. Orion Pictures Corporation.

[9] Kerr, John. 1993. A Most Dangerous Method: The Story of Jung, Freud, and Sabina Spielrein, New York: Alfred A Knopf, 1993

[10] "Homer the Vigilante." Gracie Films, 20th century Fox Television, February 20, 1994.

[11] IHME, Global Burden of Disease (2024) – with major processing by Our World in Data. "Share of population with mental health disorders" [dataset]. IHME, Global Burden of Disease, "Global Burden of Disease - Prevalence and Incidence" [original data]. Retrieved November 14, 2024, from https://ourworldindata.org/grapher/share-with-mental-and-substance-disorders

[12] McLachlan, Stacey. "45 Facebook Statistics Marketers Need to Know in 2024." Hootsuite (blog), August 2, 2024. https://blog.hootsuite.com/facebook-statistics/

[13] Mental Health: World Health Organization; 2022. Licence: CC BY-NC-SA 3.0 IGO. https://www.who.int/news-room/fact-sheets/detail/mental-health-strengthening-our-response

[14] Maslow (1943) Psychological Review 50, pp. 370-396.A Theory of Human Motivation.

[15] Jung, C. G. 1968. Psychology and Alchemy, Collected Works of C. G. Jung. Princeton, NJ: Princeton University Press.

[16] Gene, Roddenberry et al. Star Trek, the Original Series. Hollywood, Calif., CBS DVD, 2008.

[17] Nietzsche, Friedrich Wilhelm, 1844-1900. Beyond Good and Evil: Prelude to a Philosophy of the Future. London, England; New York, USA: Penguin Books, 1990.

[18] Hall, Terry. Golding, Lynval. Staples, Neville. Fun Boy Three. The Lunatics Have Taken Over the Asylum. 1981. Chrysalis Records Limited

[19] BBC. (1961–Present). Points of View. [Television series]. BBC.

[20] Lucasfilm Ltd.; 20th Century Fox. Star Wars Original Trilogy. [San Francisco]: Beverly Hills, Calif.: Lucasfilm; Twentieth Century Fox Home Entertainment, 2013.

[21] Cambridge University Press (n.d.): Term. In Cambridge Dictionary. Retrieved January 14, 2025, from https://dictionary.cambridge.org/us/dictionary/english/term

[22] Pescosolido, B. A., Halpern-Manners, A., Luo, L., & Perry, B. (2021). Trends in Public Stigma of Mental Illness in the US, 1996-2018. JAMA Network open, 4(12), e2140202. https://doi.org/10.1001/jamanetworkopen.2021.40202

[23] Farrelly, Frank. Provocative Therapy. New York: Brunner/Mazel, 1974.

[24] GBD Results Tool. In: Global Health Data Exchange [website]. Seattle: Institute for Health Metrics and Evaluation; 2019 (https://vizhub.healthdata.org/gbd-results?params=gbd-api-2019-permalink/716f37e05d94046d6a06c1194a8eb0c9, accessed 5 September 2023).

[25] Alonso J, Liu Z, Evans-Lacko S, et al. Treatment gap for anxiety disorders is global: results of the World Mental Health Surveys in 21 countries. Depress Anxiety. 2018;35(3):195–208. doi:10.1002/da.22711.

[26] Website, Nhs. "Overview - Post-traumatic Stress Disorder." nhs.uk, January 15, 2025. https://www.nhs.uk/mental-health/conditions/post-traumatic-stress-disorder-ptsd/overview/.

[27] IHME, Global Burden of Disease (2024) – with major processing by Our World in Data. "Age-standardized" [dataset]. IHME, Global Burden of Disease, "Global Burden of Disease - Mental Health Prevalence" [original data].

[28] Cohen, David; Matt Groening; Bill Oakley (2005). The Simpsons season 7 DVD commentary for the episode "Much Apu About Nothing" (DVD). 20th Century Fox.

[29] Hawkins, David R. Power vs. Force: The Hidden Determinants of Human Behavior. Hay House, 1995

[30] Coppola, Francis Ford. 1972. The Godfather. United States: Paramount Pictures

[31] McLaren JL, Zito JM, Fegert JM and Barnett ER (2024) Editorial: Psychotropic overprescribing to youth: scope of the problem, causes, and possible solutions. Front. Psychiatry 15:1418600. doi: 10.3389/fpsyt.2024.1418600

[32] Sutcliffe, A. G. (1999). Prescribing medicines for children: Major problems exist, but there are some promising developments. BMJ : British Medical Journal, 319(7202), 70. https://doi.org/10.1136/bmj.319.7202.70

[33] Ferrara, Abel. The Driller Killer. Motion Picture. 1979. Navaron Films.

[34] Deodato, Ruggero. Cannibal Holocaust. Motion Picture. 1980. F.D. Cinematografica.

[35] Raimi, Sam. The Evil Dead. Motion picture. 1981. Empire Pictures.

[36] The Big Bang Theory: Created by Chuck Lorre and Bill Prady, produced by Chuck Lorre Productions and Warner Bros. Television, 2007-2019.

[37] McLachlan, Stacey. "45 Facebook Statistics Marketers Need to Know in 2024." Hootsuite (blog), August 2, 2024. https://blog.hootsuite.com/facebook-statistics/

[38] Morecambe, Eric, and Wise, Ernie. "The Morecambe and Wise Show: Christmas Show 1971." BBC, December 25, 1971.

[39] The X-Files: Title of Television Show. 1993-2002. Fox. DVD.

[40] Sheldrake, Rupert. 2020. The Science Delusion. London. Hodder & Stoughton Ltd.

[41] Lipton, Bruce. The Biology of Belief. Santa Rosa, CA: Mountain of Love/Elite Books, 2005.

[42] Office for National Statistics (ONS), released 29 November 2022, ONS website, statistical bulletin, Religion, England and Wales: Census 2021

[43] PRRI. "2020 PRRI Census of American Religion." PRRI | at the Intersection of Religion, Values, and Public Life., August 29, 2024. https://www.prri.org/research/2020-census-of-american-religion/.

[44] YouGov. "Agree or Disagree: I enjoy giving more than receiving presents". https://www.yougov.chat/channels/daily-chat-uk/27647. Accessed January 24, 2025.

[45] Text generated by Google Gemini, Google, November. 10, 2024, https://gemini.google.com.

[46] The Matrix: Lilly Wachowski and Lana Wachowski, directors. Warner Bros., 1999.

[47] Hicks, Bill. Revelations. Directed by Chris Bould. 1993. TV special.

[48] Sausage!

About the Author

Stuart Welbourn is the author of *It's Not OK to Be Not OK* and the not-for-profit book *PTSD: A Self-Help Survival Guide*.

After being medically discharged from the Royal Navy in 1996, Stuart retrained as a psychotherapist specialising in anxiety disorders.

In 2017, Stuart earned his Master's Degree in Film, adding a fresh dynamic to his self-help endeavours by examining the role of acting and performance in personality and mental well-being.

Stuart's mission is to help some of society's most overlooked members develop levels of consciousness usually reserved for the wealthy and privileged through his writing and talks.

Discover more at stuartwelbourn.com

What's Next?

This book was just a starting point for improving mental health and raising consciousness levels. I firmly believe that one of the main reasons many advanced techniques for achieving life's desires remain elusive for so many people is due to a common factor: spending much of life in a victim mindset, often unconsciously. Once you've worked through this, I think anything is truly possible. This is why the other book I'm writing goes deeper into the secondary benefits of being a victim, the things you can do about the mindset, and what you can do to never feel like that again. It's not a miracle cure for all. I'm no narci-chologist, so I shall just say that it could significantly change the lives of some who read it. Maybe you'll be one of them? Or perhaps you'll find what you need somewhere else. I know it's a bit of a dick move to be promoting another book to you in a book you're reading, but I started writing that one first. Writing two books at the same time is probably also a good indicator that I do have ADHD, after all.

Note: I need to point out that I have started a third book since I first wrote that last sentence. Ironically, it was on the day I could have completed the first draft of this book; the evidence is surely stacking up against me!

Printed in Dunstable, United Kingdom

66272301R00087